Making Aging in Place Work

Making Aging in Place Work has been co-published simultaneously as *Journal of Housing for the Elderly,* Volume 13, Numbers 1/2 1999.

The *Journal of Housing for the Elderly* Monographic "Separates"

Below is a list of "separates," which in serials librarianship means a special issue simultaneously published as a special journal issue or double-issue *and* as a "separate" hardbound monograph. (This is a format which we also call a "DocuSerial.")

"Separates" are published because specialized libraries or professionals may wish to purchase a specific thematic issue by itself in a format which can be separately cataloged and shelved, as opposed to purchasing the journal on an on-going basis. Faculty members may also more easily consider a "separate" for classroom adoption.

"Separates" are carefully classified separately with the major book jobbers so that the journal tie-in can be noted on new book order slips to avoid duplicate purchasing.

You may wish to visit Haworth's Website at . . .

http://www.haworthpressinc.com

. . . to search our online catalog for complete tables of contents of these separates and related publications.

You may also call 1-800-HAWORTH (outside US/Canada: 607-722-5857), or Fax 1-800-895-0582 (outside US/Canada: 607-771-0012), or e-mail at:

getinfo@haworthpressinc.com

Making Aging in Place Work, edited by Leon A. Pastalan, PhD (Vol. 13, No. 1/2, 1999). *Addressing issues ranging from home modification to treatment of depression, this book will help you identify the needs of the elderly in order to offer them a comfortable and more independent life.*

Shelter and Service Issues for Aging Populations: International Perspectives, edited by Leon A. Pastalan, PhD (Vol. 12, No. 1/2, 1997). *"Provides an international perspective on meeting the housing and service needs of the elderly. The book outlines the strengths and weaknesses of different approaches, policies, and cost-effective, successful arrangements."* (Older Americans Report)

Housing Decisions for the Elderly: To Move or Not to Move, edited by Leon Pastalan, PhD (Vol. 11, No. 2, 1995). *"This insightful book thoroughly explores the crucial decisions many elderly face, and it provides a comprehensive overview of the complex problems that are associated with these decisions."* (Benyamin Schwarz, PhD, Assistant Professor, Environmental Design Department, University of Missouri)

University-Linked Retirement Communities: Student Visions of Eldercare, edited by Leon A. Pastalan, PhD, and Benyamin Schwarz (Vol. 11, No. 1, 1994). *"A masterpiece. . . . Provides one of the most comprehensive set of illustrations for integrating research-based theory with design to date. . . . The contribution this book makes to a better understanding of the multidisciplinary nature of the design process is profound."* (Ronald G. Phillips, ArchD, Director, Graduate Studies Program, Department of Environmental Design, University of Missouri-Columbia)

Congregate Housing for the Elderly: Theoretical, Policy, and Programmatic Perspectives, edited by Lenard W. Kaye, DSW, and Abraham Monk, PhD (Vol. 9, No. 1/2, 1992). *"Significant authorities present concise factual chapters about federal housing policies, services for elders, models of service assisted housing, enhanced or supported housing and 'assisted living,' and specifically, the federal congregate Housing Services Program."* (Journal of the American Geriatrics Society)

Residential Care Services for the Elderly: Business Guide for Home-Based Eldercare, edited by Doris K. Williams, PhD (Vol. 8, No. 2, 1991). *"A how-to-do-it manual for persons considering establishing a home-based business to provide residential care services for elderly people."* (Science Books & Films)

Housing Risks and Homelessness Among the Urban Elderly, edited by Sharon M. Keigher, PhD (Vol. 8, No. 1, 1991). *"A good beginning for an understanding of homelessness among older persons. . . . Useful for policymakers in their pursuit of useful and valid information that would serve to focus the* *direction of future polices and programs related to homelessness, especially among those who are older." (Educational Gerontology)*

Granny Flats as Housing for the Elderly: International Perspectives, edited by N. Michael Lazarowich, PhD (Vol. 7, No. 2, 1991). *"An informative guide to the latest experimental projects and government programs to encourage the provision of 'granny flats' or 'echo housing'-apartment or other dwelling units which are wholly or partly linked to or within a family dwelling.'' (Tony Warnes, Kings College, London)*

Optimizing Housing for the Elderly: Homes Not Houses, edited by Leon A. Pastalan, PhD (Vol. 7, No. 1, 1991). *"Especially helpful to planners and policy developers in the area of housing alternatives for the elderly. There is a clear effort to provide a range of options for professional intervention.'' (Science Books & Films)*

Aging in Place: The Role of Housing and Social Supports, edited by Leon A. Pastalan, PhD (Vol. 6, No. 1/2, 1990). *"Emphasizes the practicalities of keeping people going in independent housing.'' (British Journal of Psychiatry)*

The Retirement Community Movement: Some Contemporary Issues, edited by Leon Pastalan, PhD (Vol. 5, No. 2, 1989). *The practical implications of the research findings provided in this key volume helps readers to identify and satisfy the needs of retirement community residents.*

Lifestyles and Housing of Older Adults: The Florida Experience, edited by Leon A. Pastalan, PhD, and Marie E. Cowart, DPH, RN (Vol. 5, No. 1, 1989). *"A good introductory source for students to understand recent efforts to amalgamate living environments and service delivery systems in order to provide better care for the elderly." (Community Alternatives)*

Aging at Home: How the Elderly Adjust Their Housing Without Moving, edited by Raymond J. Struyk, PhD, and Harold M. Katsura, MCRP (Vol. 4, No. 2, 1988). *"Of value in the development of a comprehensive theory of environmental adjustment relevant regardless of age for those whom living in place has become problematic.'' (Disabilities Studies Quarterly)*

Continuing Care Retirement Communities: Political, Social, and Financial Issues, edited by Ian A. Morrison, Ruth Bennett, PhD, Susana Frisch, MA, and Barry J. Gurland, MD (Vol. 3, No. 1/2, 1986). *"Well-written and comprehensive in scope." (The Gerontologist)*

Retirement Communities: An American Original, edited by Michael E. Hunt, Allan G. Feldt, Robert W. Marans, Leon A. Pastalan, and Kathleen L. Vakalo (Vol. 1, No. 3/4, 1984). *A thorough, informative volume on retirement communities in the United States.*

Making Aging in Place Work

Leon A. Pastalan
Editor

Making Aging in Place Work has been co-published simultaneously as *Journal of Housing for the Elderly*, Volume 13, Numbers 1/2 1999.

The Haworth Press, Inc.
New York • London • Oxford

Making Aging in Place Work has been co-published simultaneously as *Journal of Housing for the Elderly,* Volume 13, Numbers 1/2 1999.

The development, preparation, and publication of this work has been undertaken with great care. However, the publisher, employees, editors, and agents of The Haworth Press and all imprints of The Haworth Press, Inc., including The Haworth Medical Press® and Pharmaceutical Products Press®, are not responsible for any errors contained herein or for consequences that may ensue from use of materials or information contained in this work. Opinions expressed by the author(s) are not necessarily those of The Haworth Press, Inc.

Cover design by Thomas J. Mayshock Jr.

The Haworth Press, Inc., 10 Alice Street, Binghamton, NY 13904-1580 USA

Library of Congress Cataloging-in-Publication Data

Making aging in place work / Leon A. Pastalan, editor.
     p. cm.
     "Co-published simultaneously as Journal of housing for the elderly, Volume 13, Numbers 1/2 1999."
     Includes bibliographical references and index.
     ISBN 0-7890-0753-3 (alk. paper)
     1. Aged–Services for–United States. 2. Aged–Government policy–United States. 3. Aged–Housing–United States. 4. Aged–Homecare–United States. I. Pastalan, Leon A., 1930- . II. Journal of housing for the elderly.
HV1461.M34 1999
362.6'0973–dc21
                                                   99-31598
                                                      CIP

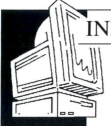

INDEXING & ABSTRACTING

Contributions to this publication are selectively indexed or abstracted in print, electronic, online, or CD-ROM version(s) of the reference tools and information services listed below. This list is current as of the copyright date of this publication. See the end of this section for additional notes.

- *Abstracts in Social Gerontology: Current Literature on Aging*

- *AgeInfo CD-ROM*

- *AgeLine Database*

- *AGRICOLA Database*

- *Applied Social Sciences Index & Abstracts (ASSIA) (Online: ASSI via Data-Star) (CDRom: ASSIA Plus)*

- *Architectural Periodicals Index*

- *BUBL Information Service: An Internet-based Information Service for the UK higher education community*

- *CINAHL (Cumulative Index to Nursing & Allied Health Literature), in print, also on CD-ROM from CD PLUS, EBSCO, and SilverPlatter, and online from CDP Online (formerly BRS), Data-Star, and PaperChase. (Support materials include Subject Heading List, Database Search Guide, and instructional video.)*

- *CNPIEC Reference Guide: Chinese National Directory of Foreign Periodicals*

- *Family Studies Database (online and CD/ROM)*

- *GEO Abstracts (GEO Abstracts/GEOBASE)*

- *Human Resources Abstracts (HRA)*

- *IBZ International Bibliography of Periodical Literature*

(continued)

- *Journal of Planning Literature/Incorporating the CPL Bibliographies*

- *Mental Health Abstracts (online through DIALOG)*

- *National Library Database on Homelessness*

- *New Literature on Old Age*

- *OT BibSys*

- *PAIS (Public Affairs Information Service) NYC*

- *Sage Urban Studies Abstracts (SUSA)*

- *Social Planning/Policy & Development Abstracts (SOPODA)*

- *Sociological Abstracts (SA)*

Special Bibliographic Notes related to special journal issues (separates) and indexing/abstracting:

- indexing/abstracting services in this list will also cover material in any "separate" that is co-published simultaneously with Haworth's special thematic journal issue or DocuSerial. Indexing/abstracting usually covers material at the article/chapter level.
- monographic co-editions are intended for either non-subscribers or libraries which intend to purchase a second copy for their circulating collections.
- monographic co-editions are reported to all jobbers/wholesalers/approval plans. The source journal is listed as the "series" to assist the prevention of duplicate purchasing in the same manner utilized for books-in-series.
- to facilitate user/access services all indexing/abstracting services are encouraged to utilize the co-indexing entry note indicated at the bottom of the first page of each article/chapter/contribution.
- this is intended to assist a library user of any reference tool (whether print, electronic, online, or CD-ROM) to locate the monographic version if the library has purchased this version but not a subscription to the source journal.
- individual articles/chapters in any Haworth publication are also available through the Haworth Document Delivery Service (HDDS).

Making Aging in Place Work

CONTENTS

ABOUT THE EDITOR

Leon A. Pastalan, PhD, is Professor of Architecture in the College of Architecture and Urban Planning at The University of Michigan. Dr. Pastalan is also Director of the National Center on Housing and Living Arrangements for Older Americans. As a researcher of long-standing in the field of environments for the elderly, he is an expert in sensory deficits, spatial behavior, and housing. Dr. Pastalan has published many books and articles resulting from his work, including *Man Environment Reference 2* (MER 2) (The University of Michigan Press, 1983), *Retirement Communities: An American Original* (The Haworth Press, Inc., 1984), *Lifestyles and Housing of Older Adults: The Florida Experience* (The Haworth Press, Inc., 1989), *Aging in Place: The Role of Housing and Social Supports* (The Haworth Press, Inc., 1990), *Optimizing Housing for the Elderly: Homes Not Houses* (The Haworth Press, Inc., 1991) and, most recently, *University-Linked Retirement Communities: Student Visions of Eldercare* (The Haworth Press, Inc., 1994), *Housing Decisions for the Elderly: To Move or Not to Move* (The Haworth Press, Inc., 1995) and *Shelter and Service Issues for Aging Populations: International Perspectives* (The Haworth Press, Inc., 1997). Dr. Pastalan is also Editor of the *Journal of Housing for the Elderly* (The Haworth Press, Inc.).

Introduction

Leon A. Pastalan

This volume focuses on some of the services that contribute to persons staying in their current living arrangement for as long as possible. These services cover a broad spectrum ranging from home modification to treatment of depression.

Clearly home modification such as installing a bathroom on the first floor where there wasn't one previously or making all rooms wheelchair accessible provides important physical supports which may facilitate remaining at home.

Living near family and friends of long standing can also provide physical and psychosocial comfort that may encourage individuals to remain where they are as studies of "naturally occurring retirement communities" point out.

An extensive discussion of a demonstration study is presented regarding support services in subsidized housing. The demonstration was geared to determine individual needs and how this impacts on aging in place. One of the needs addressed by another author is psychological counseling for residents who are depressed.

A sobering note is expressed in one of the articles which points out that what professional services providers ranging from housing to health care think is important is not necessarily what residents consider important in terms of aging in place.

What may in fact represent the ultimate measures taken to keep persons in their residence is a Homecare Suite. This is not where a health care provider comes to deliver care in a typical residential setting but is a functional nursing care unit. This nursing care module

[Haworth co-indexing entry note]: "Introduction." Pastalan, Leon A. Co-published simultaneously in *Journal of Housing for the Elderly* (The Haworth Press, Inc.) Vol. 13, No. 1/2, 1999, pp. 1-2; and: *Making Aging in Place Work* (ed: Leon A. Pastalan) The Haworth Press, Inc., 1999, pp. 1-2. Single or multiple copies of this article are available for a fee from The Haworth Document Delivery Service [1-800-342-9678, 9:00 a.m. - 5:00 p.m. (EST). E-mail address: getinfo@haworthpressinc.com].

can be temporarily installed in a garage and has many of the medical appliances and equipment necessary to support a resident in need of care on-site.

In conclusion, aging in place is perhaps one of the most important housing concepts we are concerned with currently and it appears to be creating a watershed change in terms of policy regarding housing and living arrangements and how it is played out in our society.

Adapting Rowhomes for Aging in Place: The Story of Baltimore's "Our Idea House"

Jo Fisher
Robert Giloth

SUMMARY. Aging in place strategies such as home modification have potential to enable older persons to remain in their own homes. Home modifications may also prevent home accidents and reduce the need for nursing homes. The South East Senior Housing Initiative (SESHI) in Baltimore, a coalition of housing, health care, social service, and community organizations, developed Our Idea House as a marketing tool to demonstrate how modest rowhomes could be made safer and more livable by small and large design changes. SESHI also conducted a small demonstration of how appropriate technical assistance could empower older people to make better decisions about their home environments. Reflections on the impacts of SESHI's efforts underscore the challenges facing aging in place strategies and how we need to have a better understanding of the incidence and incentives for home modification. *[Article copies available for a fee from The Haworth Document Delivery Service: 1-800-342-9678. E-mail address: getinfo@haworthpressinc.com]*

Jo Fisher is a consultant on aging and home modification issues in the Baltimore area and was formerly the Project Coordinator of the South East Senior Housing Initiative. Robert Giloth is Senior Associate at the Annie E. Casey Foundation and former Executive Director of the South East Community Organization.

The authors would like to thank the older residents of Southeast Baltimore, the SESHI steering committee, the South East Community Organization, Brian Latronico, Elizabeth Cocke, and Marci LeFevre.

A portion of this paper is based upon research collected and analyzed by Deborah A. Dougherty with the help and under the auspices of the South East Senior Housing Initiative.

[Haworth co-indexing entry note]: "Adapting Rowhomes for Aging in Place: The Story of Baltimore's 'Our Idea House.'" Fisher, Jo, and Robert Giloth. Co-published simultaneously in *Journal of Housing for the Elderly* (The Haworth Press, Inc.) Vol. 13, No. 1/2, 1999, pp. 3-18; and: *Making Aging in Place Work* (ed: Leon A. Pastalan) The Haworth Press, Inc., 1999, pp. 3-18. Single or multiple copies of this article are available for a fee from The Haworth Document Delivery Service [1-800-342-9678, 9:00 a.m. - 5:00 p.m. (EST). E-mail address: getinfo@haworthpressinc.com].

KEYWORDS. Home modification, incentives for home modification, home accidents, rowhomes, safety, livability, aging in place strategies

INTRODUCTION

The U.S. population over sixty-five is growing and, for a variety of reasons, prefers to remain in their own homes and neighborhoods, or "age in place" (Mutschler 1994). Older people frequently own their homes free and clear and thus these homes offer inexpensive housing. Homes are also repositories of, and locational access for, physical, social, and biographical meanings of place (Rowles 1993; Fogel 1992). In an aggregate sense, most older people age and retire in place, in "unplanned" senior housing rather than relocating to purpose-built senior housing or to retirement regions (Hunt and Ross 1990). That is, they stay where they are. Aging in place, however, particularly if it is to be a successful strategy for low and moderate income people, requires a wide array of human, financial, and home maintenance and modification services to enable older residents to meet their needs and preferences (Pynoos 1992; Golant 1992).

From a public policy perspective, the debate about national health care, long-term care, and "wellness" underscores the need to understand the real and potential impacts of aging in place on health-care costs and the quality of life for older people. In particular, falls in the home, which represent the fourth leading cause of death for seniors, are often a result of home environment characteristics related to stairs, bathrooms, and kitchens. The use of expensive medical procedures and the premature and unnecessary admission to nursing homes can be significantly altered by preventing falls (Moss 1992).

Modifications thought to be effective in reducing falls and other accidents include installing a bathroom on the first floor, removing scatter rugs, or utilizing grab bars. Research, however, is inconclusive about the benefit/cost of aging in place and home modification compared to nursing home costs. Moreover, there are significant challenges in achieving utilization of prevention services (e.g., counseling) by older populations before adequate evaluation results about the impacts of these services can be obtained (German 1994). Although a recent AARP survey reported that 53 percent of their sample of older people had made home modifications, the few formal studies on housing adjustment by older persons suggest that only between 2 and 10 percent of this population have made home modifications or room adjustments, and many of these changes are small (AARP 1993; Golant 1992; Rechosvsky and Newmann 1990; Struyk and Katsura 1987).

A major challenge for promoting and including home modification as a component of aging in place strategies is that it involves multiple and cross-cutting goals, systems, and actors. The challenge is how health, housing, finance and social services can be packaged to meet the distinctive needs of specific individuals, many of whom differ in terms of resources, preferences, health-care needs, and neighborhood characteristics (Golant 1992; Redfoot 1993; Newman 1993). Formula-driven programs will not work (Struyk and Katsura 1987). Many older persons also do not like to be identified or stigmatized as seniors, preferring to be empowered participants in service delivery (Cooper and Miaoulis 1988). In addition, services need to recognize the complexity, multiple participants, and the frequently prolonged life planning and decision-making for older persons.

Understanding the potential and challenges of including home modification in aging in place strategies is at a beginning stage. Very little is known about why, how often, and when older persons make adaptive modifications to their homes. The South East Senior Housing Initiative (SESHI) of Baltimore, and its "Our Idea House," provides a useful example of promoting home modifications and aging in place. It is as much a cautionary tale as it is a road map that details proven home modification and aging in place strategies. We tell the story of SESHI–its activities and impacts–as one way to gain a better understanding of the potential and limitations of home modification techniques to promote aging in place.

SESHI AND SOUTHEAST BALTIMORE

The South East Senior Housing Initiative (SESHI) is a coalition of community organizations, health-care institutions, social service agencies, senior centers, and churches that came together in 1989 with an interest in increasing housing options for older residents of southeast Baltimore (SESHI 1991). Southeast Baltimore is home to over 76,861 people, 11,854 (15.4 percent) of whom are 65 years of age and older compared to 13.99 percent for Baltimore City. Of this older population, 3,954 live alone, 3,110 have limited mobility or capacity for self care, and 2,608 have incomes below the poverty line (U.S. Census 1990). There are also a substantial number of older residents who have annual incomes in the range of the Baltimore City median, about $23,000 (U.S. Census 1990; Jubilee Baltimore 1991).

Most of these older residents live in century-old two and three story rowhouses that, in addition to requiring ongoing home maintenance and repair, are partially ill-suited to meet the physical needs of people who are becoming physically frail. Bathrooms are frequently located on the second floors; kitchens are sometimes in the basements; and most rowhomes are blessed (or cursed) with Baltimore's famed marble steps on the front exteriors. These design features are not immutable, but certainly require more than maintenance and repair levels of investment if they are to be surmounted. There are few other housing options in the community. Older residents must cope, move, or modify their homes.

SESHI believed that enabling older residents to stay in their own homes was important for community development reasons as well as being the preference of seniors. Older residents represent as high as 40 percent of the homeowners in some southeast neighborhoods and are responsible for much of the disposable income that is expended within the neighborhood commercial strips. They are "stayers," whose families have passed their homes on to succeeding generations (O'Bryant and Murray). They also perform vital social functions in the community, providing "eyes and ears," volunteering time and resources to non-profit institutions, and participating in many helping networks. SESHI members believed that intergenerational communities benefit everyone.

SESHI conducted a study, in 1990, of the housing preferences and needs of older southeast residents in order to get a better understanding of what they wanted before developing plans to increase housing options. This study included a review of census data, a survey of existing senior housing, focus groups, home interviews with home-bound seniors, prototype architectural designs, and a conference of aging in place practitioners (SESHI 1991).

Several key findings from this research shaped SESHI's thinking about aging in place strategies. First, people wanted to stay in their own homes and neighborhoods, and identified an array of support services, including help with home maintenance and chores, which they felt would make this goal easier to achieve. Second, most people were not aware of existing aging in place housing strategies and pro-grams–home maintenance, home modification, reverse equity mort-gages, and home sharing. Finally, people wanted a larger choice of housing options within the community–particularly independent liv-ing in rental housing, but also some limited forms of supported or group living.

Out of the market research emerged a consensus for SESHI action. Six recommendations were defined: (1) creation of a model home, counseling component, and resource guide on home modification; (2) expansion of home maintenance programs for seniors and a system for contractor referrals; (3) coordination and innovation of services (e.g., chore and home maintenance) to enable older residents to remain in their homes; (4) expansion of the range of senior housing options through promotion, development, and financing; (5) expansion of community organization capacity to address the needs and preferences of older residents; and (6) preservation of the long-term viability and diversity of southeast Baltimore. These recommendations set the stage for SESHI's experimental work in promoting home modification as a path to "aging in place" during the next three years.

OUR IDEA HOUSE (OIH)

SESHI decided to focus on the first recommendation of its report by acquiring and modifying an existing rowhouse. This "senior friendly" model home would show how a bathroom could be added to the first floor; and showcase equipment such as grab bars, stair lifts, higher commodes, and enhanced lighting. Guided tours would be given and visitors would have the opportunity to evaluate various products and design features in light of their own needs, preferences, and resources. Information would also be provided about the availability of products, financing techniques, contractor selection, and other related programs and services.

Word of SESHI's search for a rowhouse soon reached a private kitchen and bath contractor who offered to purchase a vacant home, modify it to SESHI's specifications, and make it available to SESHI for a nominal cost. SESHI agreed, and the contractor purchased a 100 year old, two story rowhouse. Although it was a typical rowhouse in some respects, it differed from many Baltimore rowhouses because it was built at grade level, lacked a basement, was unusually small, and had a first floor bathroom. Substantial rehabilitation was required.

As in most home designs, the SESHI house embodied many compromises. During the design process, SESHI and its advisors wavered between designing a home for people experiencing minimal impairments and for those with a range of disabilities and special needs. The final design included a first floor with a large eat-in kitchen with laundry facilities, a full, wheelchair accessible bathroom, and a closet containing the furnace and hot water heater off a living room large enough to accommodate a daybed. The second floor contained two bedrooms and a wheelchair accessible half bath. Relocating the stairs enabled the first floor design and the installation of a stairlift.

As the rehabilitation neared completion, it became apparent that references to a "model home" were leading to unrealistic expectations. It had cost nearly $100,000 to purchase and renovate the home according to the contractor—and that was way out of reach of most southeast Baltimore residents. Therefore, SESHI changed the concept to a house of ideas and named the home "Our Idea House" (OIH). The renamed house was appropriate because OIH visitors also contributed their ideas about what was left out, what did not work, and what would work better. It was a learning environment for everyone. Over 2,000 people visited Our Idea House during the sixteen months that it was open, from southeast Baltimore, other city neighborhoods, the metropolitan area, and nearby states.

TECHNICAL ASSISTANCE FOR HOME MODIFICATION

After several months of OIH operation, it became apparent that southeast residents needed and wanted assistance in implementing the ideas they gathered while visiting OIH. They often came back for a second and third visit, sometimes with family and friends. They had specific questions. In response to their questions and aided with a small grant, SESHI developed a formal process of technical assistance for southeast residents who, after visiting OIH, expressed a desire to modify their homes.

SESHI's theory of technical assistance was that older people should control the process as much as possible, with help from family or other advisors. Upon invitation, the SESHI coordinator visited seniors in their homes to learn what changes they were considering, and to perform a home audit to see if there were other changes which might enhance safety and independence. The home audit always began with the area of concern identified by the senior and then, with permission of the senior, moved on to include entryways, stairs, kitchen, bathroom, passageways, laundry facilities, lighting, flooring coverings, and fire safety. After the home visit, staff prepared a menu of possible ways to enhance safety and comfort, unique to each senor, for the senior to review.[1] If the senior chose specific options, SESHI was able to provide (through a network of staff, volunteers and consultants) architectural design, home assessment by occupational therapists, cost estimates and, if necessary, assistance in identifying funding sources.

Thirteen persons (10 females living alone, one male living alone, and one couple) ranging in age from 62 to 82 availed themselves of SESHI's technical assistance during the first 12 months that it was offered. In six cases, the main concern was modifying or relocating the bathroom; in four cases, it was relocating the stairs or installing a stairlift; and in two cases it was modifying the kitchen. Of the 12 cases, one resulted in a total home modification with a new staircase, a bathroom installed on the first floor, and a new efficient kitchen design including a laundry; three people modified their bathrooms; one person installed a stairlift; one person modified her kitchen and installed additional lighting; two persons died before taking any action; one decided not to do anything; and three cases remained open.

Piecing Together Resources

One of the more complex cases involved the installation of a stairlift in the home of a 64 year old woman on medical disability who suffered from multiple health problems including asthma and severe arthritis. She had an income of $422 per month from Social Security and received medical and fuel assistance. Her four room home, which had been in the family for over 70 years, had a very steep cross stairs. Climbing the stairs caused her great pain. The home audit also revealed a need for grab bars in the bathroom.

SESHI referred her to the Maryland Division of Rehabilitation Services which, under its Independent Living Program, agreed to install

---

1. SESHI later developed *Staying Home: Ways for Older Americans to Make Their Homes Fit Their Needs,* a video with resource and guide booklet, which reviews an array of home modifications and resources for older adults.

the stairlift, toilet and grab bars free of charge In preparing the installation, however, they determined that the grade in the stairwell, which they calculated to be 54 degrees, was too great to safely install a stairlift. In her disappointment over that setback, she declined their offer to install the toilet and grab bars in the bathroom.

At the woman's request, SESHI obtained a second opinion from a local stairlift vendor. After examining the stairwell, the contractor determined that a stairlift could be used safely, and he agreed to rehabilitate and install a donated stairlift in her home at a reduced price. But because even this cost was too high for her fixed income, SESHI worked to identify other funding sources. Ultimately, her church provided an electrician, the local Arthritis Foundation made a small donation, and a local foundation which provides last resort funding for home modifications provided the balance. Grab bars were installed in the bathroom using similar community resources.

An Enterprising Couple Makes Small Changes

A second case involved a couple who visited OIH and decided that they would also benefit from a stairlift. The woman was 77 years old and reported she was in good health. Her 82 year old husband had suffered several heart attacks and mini-strokes; he reported frequent numbness in his right leg and what he called "near falls." Both expressed concern about falling on the stairs or in the bathtub.

During the home audit, SESHI identified several unsafe areas in the home and suggested installing a stairlift in the stairwell most frequently used, installing handrails on both sides of all three stairwells, installing two sets of grab bars in the bathroom (each person had specific needs), removing many of the ubiquitous scatter rugs found throughout the house, and rearranging furniture which protruded into pathways.

The menu of recommendations to the couple advised limiting the use of the basement studio, installing a stairlift and handrails, removing scatter rugs, installing grab bars in the bathroom, and rearranging furniture. SESHI also recommended that they invite an occupational therapist into the home to perform a more detailed assessment. Within a day of receiving the list, the couple had implemented several of the recommendations, although they decided against the stairlift because they thought the cost was excessive.

Some Houses Just Don't Adapt

A third case involved a newly-retired 62 year old woman in excellent health. In planning for her future housing needs, she was considering an array of independent living options: a continuing care community in another city; relocating to another home in Baltimore to be closer to family; and modifying her home to accommodate what she anticipated to be her future needs.

Her current home is a thirteen foot wide, two story rowhouse with narrow transverse interior stairwells and with the only bathroom at the back of the second floor. There are five stairs on the outside at the front and rear; and there is no direct access to an alley or street from the rear. She feels that the day is coming when she will not be able to safely use the stairs to either the basement or second floor.

Anticipating her future needs, she requested help from SESHI in examining how a larger bathroom might be built on the second floor and how the stairs could be modified to allow for the installation of a stair lift should she ever need it. At SESHI's request, consultants developed designs and cost estimates. At first, the $25,000 estimate for these changes seemed reasonable, but later, when she considered the potential costs of other modifications (such as an exterior lift at the front of the house), she decided that it was not cost effective to modify her home. She decided to explore the possibility of purchasing another home in the neighborhood with a more flexible design.

EVALUATING OUR IDEA HOUSE
AND HOME MODIFICATION

Initiating, completing and operating Our Idea House (OIH) was a "labor of love" for SESHI and its many friends and supporters. OIH required a great deal of energy and resources for marketing, attracting and training volunteers, operating expenses, and for maintaining organizational interest. After one year of operating OIH, SESHI members began to ask: Are visitors to OIH making home modifications? Are we reaching the right people? Is OIH the most effective way to communicate our message about home modification? These questions resonated with the everyday experience of operating the house: fewer people seemed interested in making home modifications than was expected.

SESHI also recognized that, in addition to the number of home modifications being made, there were other ways the impact of operating OIH might be measured: how the hundreds of professionals in the aging field who had visited OIH were using the information they gathered there; the effect of the OIH experience on state and local aging programs and policies; the fit between OIH and regional and national home modification programs; the fit between SESHI and local health care institutions; and the effect of exposure to OIH on the decision-making processes of older residents and their families. In the end, and with assistance of a research intern from the University of Baltimore, SESHI began by trying to understand the reactions and changed behaviors, if any, of older residents who had visited OIH.

SESHI phone-surveyed a sample of 344 older residents of metropolitan Baltimore who had visited OIH prior to July, 1993. Questions focussed on why respondents visited OIH, what they liked and disliked about OIH, whether they had made home modifications or intended to, why not if they had not made modifications, demographic characteristics (including income), and who helped them make home modification decisions. Responses were obtained from 227 OIH visitors, a 70 percent completion rate for those contacted. In general, people were quite willing to answer questions: they had enjoyed their OIH visit and felt strongly about the issues.

The majority of the respondents to the OIH survey were between 66-75, mostly white women, married or widowed, in good health, and homeowners. Almost 16 percent had received college degrees, and median household income was between $15-29,999. Although almost two-thirds of those interviewed had visited OIH out of curiosity, the balance of people said that they planned to make renovations, experienced limitations in activity or problems in their own homes, or were planning home changes for others. They identified the kitchen, bathroom, or specific features in each, as the most useful parts of OIH.

Thirty-two of those surveyed (14 percent) had made modifications to their homes at the time of the survey while seventy-five, or 33 percent, planned to make changes in the future. Most of the changes were relatively inexpensive: installation of grab bars and handles, raised outlets, hand rails, and shower seats. Several, however, had renovated bathrooms and kitchens. Most respondents who said they planned future changes did not specify the types of changes they would make. Twenty-seven percent did say that they would modify their bathrooms or install chair lifts.

Whether home modifications were made or not was strongly associated with the income, education, and location outside of southeast Baltimore. Those making home modifications more frequently had incomes of $16,000 or more and had graduated from high school. Those who indicated a problem with their current home were also more likely to make modifications. Living outside of southeast Baltimore typically meant living in a higher income city or suburban neighborhood. The influence of income, education, and location were even stronger for those who planned future home modifications (Dougherty 1993).

What the findings of the OIH survey show is that people take time to make decisions about changing their home environments, make small changes first, are more likely to make changes when they are experiencing problems in their homes, and rely upon advice from siblings and professionals. Financial constraints affect the receptivity of people to home modification ideas; and consequently, lower income seniors are less likely to make home modifications.

WHAT SESHI LEARNED FROM TECHNICAL ASSISTANCE

The technical assistance cases contain many important lessons. Southeast's older residents are proud, hard-working, and frugal. Many of their homes have been handed down through three generations. SESHI found these cultural and economic givens were interwoven with other critical factors such as coping mechanisms, family support, communication, and expectations about community resources. The result is a complex decision-making process.

Several residents live in homes where furniture is arranged much as it had been in their parent's day. SESHI worked with residents who remember parents crawling up steep steps when they could no longer walk up them, and who now, themselves crawl up those same stairs. Residents spoke with pride of how bathrooms were built on the back of the second story after World War II. Modifying these homes may upset personal histories.

Many of SESHI's seniors appeared to seek assistance only when their coping mechanisms no longer addressed their needs. Some people, for example, had abandoned the use of parts of their homes.

One woman crawled up and down the basement stairs to shelves where she kept extra food items. One man ate his meals out of his home when his heart condition precluded using the stairs to access his basement kitchen. Another woman was housebound because she could not use the outside stairs.

There are a number of reasons why older southeast residents cope with environments which do not support their physical needs. They may deny, ignore, or be desensitized to the deficiencies of their housing; their housing problems may pale compared to their other problems or their familiarity with their housing, deficient as it may be, may lend them security or confidence (Golant 1992). Whatever the reason, in ten of the twelve cases in which SESHI provided technical assistance, home assessments uncovered deficiencies beyond those which the resident had identified. Deficiencies included faulty electrical systems, lack of handrails and grab bars, potentially dangerous furniture placement, and poor lighting.

Support from family and friends was important; it was evident in nine of the twelve cases. Of the six cases in which modifications were completed, all had active family support. This support was often financial as well as emotional.

Communication was another important factor. Older people typically receive conflicting messages from different sources: children telling them to move or telling them that their problems are psychological; health care professionals with little or no understanding of the home conditions of their patients; and contractors who do not understand the needs and preferences of older people. Facilitating communication between all parties became an integral part of SESHI's technical assistance.

Many older people believed public programs either existed or should exist to help make home modifications. Those who did have savings did not want to spend their own resources on home modification; they planned to bequeath these assets to heirs–in spite of the present impact on their quality of life.

Only one person agreed to borrow money. She considered a reverse equity mortgage only to find out that the closing costs would equal the amount of money she wanted to borrow. Though she was income eligible for a low-interest, deferred city loan, the long processing time for the loan prompted her children to pay for and install a shower in a first floor laundry room rather than borrow money to add a more costly bathroom on the first floor.

SESHI also learned that the process of home modification can be overwhelming to the older person. Even the advice of professionals can be overwhelming. In one case, an older woman asked for help in determining how a bathroom could be installed in her basement, the site of her kitchen and family room. Because her basement was a jungle of pipes and ducts, an architect was asked to judge the feasibility of this proposal. He recommended locating the bathroom on the first floor and moving the kitchen from the basement to the first floor. She broke into tears after seeing his plan; it was too much change. Only months later did she reopen the issue with SESHI. In another case, an older woman had to vacate her home for an extended period while it was being modified, causing her and her family considerable distress.

For some southeast Baltimore homes and homeowners, home modification is simply not a cost-effective option. Many others only considered home modification after they were in crisis–and frequently modifications could not be performed in time to meet their needs.

CONCLUSION

The SESHI experience offers a rich example of an urban, working class community attempting to develop an "aging in place" network and strategy. This community neither faced the difficult housing and neighborhood conditions of many low-income, older people of color, nor did it have the equity base of higher income seniors that could be converted into usable resources for home modification. Nevertheless, SESHI's accomplishments, although modest, involved innovative approaches to planning, collaboration, marketing, and community education about the potential of small and large home modifications. In the process, older residents of Southeast Baltimore and beyond were enabled to make more informed choices about their homes and neighborhoods.

But pursuing an aging in place strategy also presented challenges for SESHI. Much is not known about aging in place and home modification, in particular the effectiveness of different strategies related to different senior cohorts. Four areas of concern and learning emerged from the SESHI experience: aging in place strategies, cost effectiveness, collaborations, and national networking. Reflecting on these challenges is useful as one guide to future research, program development and policy innovation about aging in place strategies.

The first concern is that aging in place information, techniques, and resources are useful and necessary but are not the whole story. Showcasing home modifications, whether in a physical structure such as Our Idea House or in slide shows, videos, or displays, enables consumers to process complex information in a realistic manner. Information, however, is not enough to help homeowners with modest incomes age in place; they need access to counseling and funding mechanisms (appropriate loans, subsidies, and tax credits) and emotional support during the decision-making process.

SESHI discovered that many older people, particularly moderate income, working-class people in their 70s and 80s, did not want to make home modifications. In their minds, they would rather cope, save their money, and leave inheritances for their children. Several implications flow from this finding. On the one hand, at some point these seniors may require home-based services or other senior housing options such as independent rental housing. On the other hand, because of the slow returns of marketing in neighborhoods such as southeast Baltimore it may make sense to market home modification and aging in place to a younger cohort of people now approaching retirement, many of whom may live in the so-called "graying suburbs."

The second concern involves the benefit/cost of helping older people modify their homes so as to prevent falls and other accidents which might lead to hospitalization and/or institutionalization. Collaborative research among practitioners in the fields of geriatrics, public health, and senior housing should develop reliable data on the benefits and costs of home modifications, and how these compare with other strategies. Research should not only evaluate the impact of more expensive home modifications such as stair lifts and accessible bathrooms, but more importantly, should examine smaller environmental changes such as home assessments, grab bars and the removal of safety hazards like scatter rugs and ill-placed furniture.

The third concern is the promotion of collaboration in the delivery of services to promote aging in place. SESHI, as a network of diverse institutions and professions, learned a great deal about the need to draw upon many resources to promote aging in place. For SESHI, the potential of collaboration was amply demonstrated during its research phase, in designing and operating Our Idea House, and in providing technical assistance. But there were also limitations: home modification services needed to be better linked to key actors in the lives of older people. Four such actors have this potential: (1) the health delivery system for older adults; (2) corporations offering benefit packages for children who frequently are involved in decision-making with their parents; (3) civic and religious institutions; (4) social welfare organizations; and (5) private contractors and home repair centers.

In many respects the most promising linkage is with the health care system. A case management process that would link health care, home modification, and home-based services in addition to home-care has the potential to improve quality of life and reduce costs. There are several models for redesigning the system: insurance-based continuing care communities on the high income end; and Medicaid-based programs for the frail elderly.

The fourth concern is to improve collaboration among organizations across the nation which have developed or are planning home modification models and programs. This has been partially achieved for home maintenance and repair services for older people. The time is right for national networking of home modification projects, lessons, and experts. SESHI learned, as it progressed with its Our Idea House and technical assistance program, of projects such as the Hartford House–a portable model developed by the ITT Hartford Insurance Group, The Adaptable Home developed in Maryland by the National Association of Home Builders, the Friendly Home developed in California by Lewis Homes, and of Jon Pynoos' directory of home modification programs. A positive sign in this regard is that the Housing Accessibility Institute of the National Association of Homebuilders recently held a national conference which dealt with many of the issues with which SESHI has grappled.

Older people want to age in place, in their homes and in their neighborhoods. Many are already doing so, but at times at a great cost to themselves and the community at large. Aging in place strategies, such as those designed and pursued by the South East Senior Housing Initiative (SESHI), are important not only because of the people they served but also because of the lessons that have been learned.

REFERENCES

American Association of Retired Persons (AARP). (1993). *Understanding senior housing for the 1990's.* Washington D.C.

Cooper, Phillip D. and Miaoulis, George. (1988). Altering corporate strategic criteria to reflect the changing environment: the role of life satisfaction and the growing senior market. *California Management Review,* 31, 87-97.

Dougherty, Deborah D. (1993). *Impact assessment of our idea house.* Unpublished manuscript. University of Baltimore, Department of Sociology, Baltimore.

Fogel, Barry S. (1992). The psychological aspects of staying at home. *Generations* 16, 15-19.

German, Pearl S. (1994). The meaning of prevention for older people: changing common perceptions. *Generations* 18, 28-32.

Golant, S.M. (1984). *A place to grow old.* New York: Columbia University Press.

Golant, S.M. (1992). *Housing America's elderly: many possibilities/few choices.* Newbury Park: Sage Publications.

Hunt, Michael E., and Ross, Leonard E. (1990). Naturally occurring retirement communities: A multiattribute examination of desirability factors. *Gerontologist* 30, 667-674.

Jubilee Baltimore. (1990). *Market study for Messiah Lutheran senior housing.* Baltimore: Jubilee Baltimore.

Moss, Anne B. (1992). Are the elderly safe at home? *Journal of Community Health Nursing.* 13-19.

Mutchler, Phyllis. Where elders live. *Generations* 16 7-14.

Newman, Sandra J. (1993). Comment on long-term care reform and the role of housing finance. *Housing Policy Debate* 4(4):551-564.

O'Bryant, Shirley L. (1983). The subjective value of home to older homeowners. *Journal of Housing for the Elderly* 1, 29-43.

Pynoos, Jon. (1990). *National directory of home modification and repair programs.* Los Angeles: University of California, Long Term Care National Resource Center.

Pynoos, Jon. (1992). Strategies for home modification and repair. *Generations,* 16, 21-25.

Redfoot, Donald L. (1993). Long-term care reform and the role of housing finance. *Housing Policy Debate* 4(4): 497-538.

Reschovsky, James D. and Newman, Sandra J. (1990). Adaptations for independent living by older frail households. *Gerontologist,* 30, 543-552.

Rowles, Graham D. (1993). Evolving images of place in aging and "aging in place." *Generations,* 17, 65-70.

South East Senior Housing Initiative (SESHI). (1991). *Meeting the housing preferences and needs of the older residents in south east Baltimore City.* Baltimore: SESHI.

Struyk, Raymond J. and Katsure, Harold M. (1987). Aging at home: How the elderly adjust their housing without moving. *Journal of Housing for the Elderly,* 4, 1-175.

U.S. Census. (1990). *Census of population.* Washington D.C.: U.S. Department of Commerce.

Varady, D.P. (1984). Determinants of interest in senior housing among the community resident elderly. *Gerontologist,* 24, 392-395.

Rural Naturally Occurring Retirement Communities: A Community Assessment Procedure

Linda J. Marshall
Michael E. Hunt

SUMMARY. An attempt was made to develop a diagnostic tool that communities could use to determine what type of naturally occurring retirement community (NORC) they are or could most likely become. Census data were obtained for 64 cities, townships, and villages in rural Wisconsin. These communities were classified as either Amenity, Bi-Focal, or Convenience NORCs on the basis of a previous survey of 907 residents. A stepwise discriminant analysis was then conducted on the Census variables using NORC type as the criterion variable. The resultant function used four Census variables and was successful in classifying 59.68% of Amenity, Bi-Focal, and Convenience NORCs. When Bi-Focal NORCs were eliminated from the analysis, one variable dropped out as a discriminator. However, three additional variables were significant discriminators. The resultant function classified 100% of Amenity and Convenience NORCs successfully. Implications for community planning are discussed. *[Article copies available for a fee from The Haworth Document Delivery Service: 1-800-342-9678. E-mail address: getinfo@ha worthpressinc.com]*

Linda J. Marshall, PhD, is Assistant Professor, Department of Child & Family Studies and Michael E. Hunt, MRCP, ArchD, is Professor and Chair, Department of Environment, Textiles and Design and Associate Director for Education, UW Institute on Aging, both at the University of Wisconsin-Madison.

[Haworth co-indexing entry note]: "Rural Naturally Occurring Retirement Communities: A Community Assessment Procedure." Marshall, Linda J., and Michael E. Hunt. Co-published simultaneously in *Journal of Housing for the Elderly* (The Haworth Press, Inc.) Vol. 13, No. 1/2, 1999, pp. 19-34; and: *Making Aging in Place Work* (ed: Leon A. Pastalan) The Haworth Press, Inc., 1999, pp. 19-34. Single or multiple copies of this article are available for a fee from The Haworth Document Delivery Service [1-800-342-9678, 9:00 a.m. - 5:00 p.m. (EST). E-mail address: getinfo@haworthpressinc.com].

KEYWORDS. Naturally Occurring Retirement Communities (NORCs), Amenity, Bi-Focal and Convenience as NORC types, diagnostic tool for classification, implications for community planning

INTRODUCTION

A number of researchers have suggested the economic value of attracting older migrants to rural communities. However, few methods are available to allow communities to assess their merits and organize systematic efforts to attract older residents. This research represents preliminary efforts at developing a diagnostic tool that could be used by community planners. Presumably, if a community could accurately assess its potential as a retirement destination and predict the type of retirees it would be likely to attract, more precise development and marketing plans could be instituted. This would potentially reduce the risk of costly planning errors and allow communities to meet the needs of current and future residents more effectively.

Overview

Naturally occurring retirement communities, or NORCs, are places that house a high percentage of older residents even though they were not expressly designed for that purpose. NORCs can assume many forms, such as apartment or condominium developments, neighborhoods, small towns, or rural areas. Furthermore, an area can become a NORC for a variety of reasons, including older residents moving to the area, existing residents aging in place, and younger residents moving away from the area. As will be discussed subsequently, fostering the development of a NORC can have substantial positive impacts on the community as a whole. A community that can attract older retirees is also likely to be able to maintain residents aging in place and provide incentives for younger residents to remain in the community.

Economic Implications

While the economic gains from retirement income are readily observable in Florida and the Sun Belt states, the implications for other states are often overlooked. In this research, we focused on rural NORCs in Wisconsin, a state not typically thought of as a retirement destination. Despite that prevailing bias, elderly migration has had significant impacts on elderly population growth, especially in particular parts of the state. For example, while the state as a whole experienced a 20 percent growth in the elderly population between 1970 and 1980, one-fifth of Wisconsin counties experienced growth of at least 30 percent (Wisconsin Department of Development 1984). Additionally, seven of Wisconsin's 10 fastest growing counties in the 1970s were also among the top 10 in percentage increase in elderly population. Most of the counties with high elderly growth rates were rural, with recreational amenities that attracted elderly migrants (Guhleman and Slesinger 1984). Many of the retirees to these communities had previously vacationed in the area prior to retirement (Voss and Fuguitt 1979).

Although we have restricted our current efforts to Wisconsin, the same living pattern has been observed at both the regional and national levels. In the Upper Great Lakes region of Michigan, Minnesota, and Wisconsin, one-third or more of all households in rural areas are headed by persons 65 years of age or older (Wisconsin Department of Development 1984). At the national level, the elderly led a movement toward rural areas beginning in the 1950s and increasing through the 1970s (Fuguitt and Tordella 1980; Heaton, Clifford, and Fuguitt 1981). The most noticeable migration pattern found across rural counties was the propensity of the elderly to move to areas rich in environmental and recreational amenities. This resulted in an infusion of new life into many rural areas, in some cases after long histories of decline.

The future of retirement migration is addressed by Fuguitt and Bealle (1993) who predict that retirement-age migration to rural areas will not increase during the 1990s because, in that decade, the small birth cohorts of the 1930s will enter their 60s. However, these authors contend that, after the year 2000, there will be an influx of people to both metropolitan and rural retirement destinations as the "baby boomers" reach retirement age. Thus, community assessment tools that allow communities to document and capitalize on their strengths will allow planners to compete more successfully for a limited number of current retirees while preparing to meet the future needs of increasing numbers of elderly migrants.

Community Benefits

Many municipalities have noticed the growing number of older people moving to rural towns and the economic resources they represent. For example, Hot Springs, Arkansas, received national attention recently when the city hired a full-time staff person to recruit older persons to become residents. Reports have also indicated that rural communities whose economies are based on retirees have outpaced other communities in per capita income growth (Richards 1988). Rural NORCs have benefited from their elderly residents in several ways, some of which are discussed below.

Infusion of Retiree Income

In many rural communities, government transfer payments to older residents (e.g., social security) are a major contribution to the county's economic base. For example, in 1984, money from these sources accounted for between 42.8 and 60.7 percent of resident income in the ten Wisconsin counties with the highest proportion of older persons. For the state as a whole, these sources represented only 32.1 percent of resident income (U.S. Bureau of Economic Analysis 1986). Furthermore, national evidence suggests that retirement income represents a substantial and growing source of personal income (Summers and Hirschl 1985; Bently 1988) that is playing an increasing role over time in the economic base of rural areas (Briggs and Rees, 1982).

Stimulation of Local Economy

Li and MacLean (1989) investigated the effects of the elderly population on small towns in Saskatchewan. They found that larger increases in the elderly population were associated with greater demands on services offered by the community and greater retail sales, further stimulating the small-town economy. Consistent with these findings, service industries were the main source of employment growth in rural areas between 1962 and 1978, with service industries outpacing goods-producing industries by 3.7 million jobs (Hirschl and Summers, 1985).

Retiree spending in the local economy creates a demand for goods and services by improving the demand/supply ratio. When this ratio becomes more favorable for investment and employment, capital and labor often follow, stimulating growth and attracting people to the area (Hirschl and Summers, 1985). For example, Smith and his colleagues (Smith, Hackbart, and van Veen 1981) estimated that, in Kentucky, one new job resulted from each $4425 of transfer income and that less than $4000 of social security payments was sufficient to create a job in rural counties. Retirees are particularly beneficial for the local economy because they tend to spend a greater percentage of their income on local businesses and services than do younger residents (Harmston 1979). Furthermore, older heads of households tend to maintain this spending advantage until they reach particularly advanced age (Boehm and Pond 1976).

A further way that retirees can stimulate the local economy is through the multiplier effect. The multiplier effect refers to the way in which monetary contributions from older residents assume greater value as they circulate through the community system. Siegal and Leuthold (1992) explain that spending by retirees flows into the local economy as older residents buy goods and services from firms and individuals in the community. This flow of payments generates income and employment for local residents. In addition, sales and property taxes flow to local governments, allowing them to provide services such as education and police protection. Subsequently, increases in income and employment create a ripple effect through the economy when the income is spent on other goods and services and sales and property taxes are collected. Thus, the economic and fiscal impacts of retiree spending are multiplied by successive rounds of spending and tax collection.

Enhanced Health Care System

A third benefit of older residents is the health care jobs they produce. In a study of largely rural northwest Wisconsin, Erikson and Huddleston (1975) found that health care was a leading sector of employment growth, even for cities with populations of less than 5000 people. They also noted that rural areas in Wisconsin have received a substantial amount of federal funds for the development of health care facilities. To the extent that a concentration of retirees in the local system creates a greater demand for these services and induces local expansion, more jobs will be created. Furthermore, there is evidence to suggest that a substantial increase in Medicare patients can stimulate the health care economy and attract a number of new, young physicians to the area (Haas and Crandall 1988). Because both the number and type of physicians are increased, the entire community benefits.

Clean Industry

One concern often voiced regarding elderly residents is that they place an excessive strain on the service sector of the community. However, Longino and Crown (1989) argue that elderly migrants are, at least initially, not only beneficial to the community, but also no burden to the community. They found that older migrants use few public services and that their medical care is largely paid for by Medicare transfers from the federal government or private insurance. The taxes generated by the infusion of retiree income substantially offset the public costs. Indeed, Fagan (1988) refers to elderly migration as a "retirement industry" that boosts the local economy and increases the tax base. He argues that large investments in the infrastructure or government tax abatements are not required to realize these benefits. What results is an industry that does not pollute or destroy the environment, but that increases the number of volunteers and contributors while benefiting churches. In short, Fagan argues that the retirement industry is an advantageous addition to areas seeking economic development.

Summary of Benefits

In summary, it appears that retirees represent a large potential for economic growth, especially for rural communities. Furthermore, these benefits can typically be realized without negative impacts on the service sector or the environment. We thus began this research with the assumption that communities would largely be in favor of recruiting more elderly residents. What we explored was how a community might best go about luring retirees to the vicinity, and the type of retirees an area might most reasonably expect to attract. Details of that approach are outlined below.

A Typology of Rural NORCs

Do all retirees want the same things from a community? The Wisconsin Rural NORC study (Hunt, Marshall, and Merrill, 1993) was one of the few studies to determine whether rural NORCs represent specialized retirement destinations that could be differentiated on the basis of the characteristics of the older migrants they attract and the community attributes older migrants find attractive.[1] Most prior studies have focused on differences among migrants, not among destination communities. In contrast, this research identified three types of rural NORCs: (a) Amenity NORCs, (b) Bi-Focal NORCs, and (c) Convenience NORCs. Differences among the NORC types were based on the attributes of the NORCs and the extent to which migrants were seeking either amenities or assistance.

According to Hunt et al. (1993), Amenity NORCs characteristically attract younger, healthier, and more active retirees who typically move to an area to escape an urban lifestyle and enjoy the natural environment. Retirees to Amenity NORCs tend to move from further away, are drawn by natural amenities, and tend to live near lakes or in the woods. These migrants are often seasonal residents prior to retirement and are less likely to have family ties in the area. At least initially, older people moving to Amenity NORCs are not concerned about their proximity to town-based services.

In contrast, Bi-Focal NORCs tend to attract retirees who are seeking natural amenities but who wish to retain proximity to friends and family. Transportation services and accessibility of the area are particularly important to older residents in these communities. Furthermore, these residents tend to be visited more often than residents of other NORC types, with children and grandchildren making up the largest share of visitors. These migrants share their desire for a rural lifestyle and the importance they place on community features with residents of Amenity NORCs. However, they also share their focus on roots in the area with Convenience NORCs.

Finally, Convenience NORCs tend to attract local people who are moving from one rural area to another nearby community. These people often have lower incomes and less education. They move to be close to relatives, because of recent widowhood, or because of a need to be closer to town-based services such as health care. Bentley and Saupe (1989) also note that Convenience NORCs tend to attract retired farmers. Those who move to Convenience NORCs are often not attracted to natural amenities because they already live in rural areas. These movers may also find Amenity NORCs unaffordable. A Convenience NORC allows older migrants to benefit from a socially sup-

1. This research was part of the Wisconsin Rural NORC Study directed by Michael E. Hunt and John L. Merrill, and was supported by grant number N311 from the University of Wisconsin Agricultural Experiment Station.

portive and convenient environment while living independently in an age-segregated setting.

In summary, large numbers of older people seem to be attracted to certain rural areas. Rural areas, in turn, are increasingly recognizing the benefits of attracting and retaining older residents. However, making plans to meet the needs of a rural community's older residents is complicated by the fact that rural NORCs differ significantly on several dimensions. The ability to assess what type of NORC a rural community might be would assist residents and governing officials in making plans to meet the needs of older migrants. Such an assessment would also allow planners to preserve or accentuate the attractive attributes of the area.

Research Objectives

In the Wisconsin Rural NORC Study discussed above (Hunt et al., 1993), a lengthy survey instrument was used to assess the characteristics and beliefs of a random sample of older residents living in 16 rural NORCs in Wisconsin. While that research resulted in a useful typology and a helpful assessment of the communities involved, it did not provide the means whereby other communities could derive benefit. Rather than suggesting that each community should embark on its own survey research, we undertook this project to identify a simple tool whereby a community could determine what type of NORC it was or could most likely become using pre-existing data. We also sought further validation for the original NORC typology.

METHOD

Sample

The sample in Hunt et al. (1993) was obtained by randomly sampling residents over the age of 65 within zip codes that had been identified as housing a high percentage of older residents. To approximate this area in the current research, a township or village was included in the sample if more than half of its area was contained within that zip code. This resulted in a sample of 62 cities, towns, and villages contained within 16 zip code areas. Data from the 1990 Census of Population and Housing was then collected on all 62 communities.

Variables of Interest

The grouping variable in the analysis was the NORC type (Amenity, Bi-Focal, or Convenience) of the zip code, based on earlier findings by Hunt et al. (1993). All communities that fell within a particular zip code were given the same NORC code. This resulted in a sample of 17 Amenity NORCs, 36 Bi-Focal NORCs, and 9 Convenience NORCs. Related variables were selected based on prior research findings, intuitive appeal, and availability in the Census data base. In total, 27 variables were selected and grouped as shown in Table 1.

RESULTS

The first goal was to ascertain which of the variables were significantly influenced by type of NORC. Of the original 27 variables, we determined that only those variables that demonstrated significant differences among the group means or that produced significant correlations with NORC type would be eligible for inclusion in the discriminant analysis. One-way analyses of variance were conducted for each variable using the three levels of NORC as the categorical variable. When significant F values were obtained, the Scheffe procedure was used to determine which means differed significantly from one another. Only six of the 27 analyses yielded significant mean squares. In each case, the Scheffe procedure also produced significant mean differences. An additional six variables produced significant correlations with NORC type. Thus, 12 variables were entered into the subsequent sequential analysis. Census items varying significantly across NORCs are shown in Table 2.

As the subscripts in Table 2 indicate, Amenity NORCs had significantly higher vacancy rates than did either Bi-Focal NORCs or Convenience NORCs. Both Convenience NORCs and Bi-Focal NORCs had a higher percentage of residents who were born in Wisconsin. In terms of industry, both Convenience and Bi-Focal NORCs had a higher percentage of workers employed in forestry and agriculture than did Amenity NORCs. In contrast, Amenity NORCs had a higher percentage of workers employed in construction than did Bi-Focal NORCs. Finally, Bi-Focal NORCs had a higher percentage of workers employed in transportation than did Amenity NORCs.

TABLE 1. Census Variables Preliminarily Selected for Discriminant Analysis

A.   Income Variables

1.	Median Household Income
2.	Per Capita Income
3.	Per Capita Retirement Income
4.	Per Capita Public Assistance Income
5.	Per Capita Social Security Income

B.   Resident Variables

6.	Population
7.	% Over 50
8.	% Over 65
9.	% Born in Wisconsin
10.	% Born in the Midwest
11.	% (25+) College Graduates
12.	% (25+) Less than Ninth Grade
13.	% (Males 15+) Widowed
14.	% (Females 15+) Widowed
15.	% (5+) Same House in 1985
16.	% (5+) Same County in 1985

C.   Housing Variables

17.	Median House Value
18.	% Vacant
19.	Rent–% of Gross Income

D.   Industry Variables

20.	% Employed in Forestry and Agriculture
21.	% Employed in Construction
22.	% Employed in Transportation
23.	% Employed in Retail Sales
24.	% Employed in Insurance and Real Estate
25.	% Employed in Entertainment
26.	% Employed in Health Care
27.	% Employed in Education

TABLE 2. Census Variables Varying Significantly Across NORCs or Correlating with NORC

Variable	Amenity	NORC Bi-Focal	Convenience	
Household Inc.				
M	20,616.06	22,195.44	24,716.89	$r = .30$
SD	3,229.46	4,192.24	5,126.90	$p < .05$
% Vacant				
M	55.53_{ab}	34.11_a	22.78_b	$F = 8.61$
SD	21.25	21.70	19.88	$p < .001$
Ret. Income				
M	832.71_a	530.31_a	476.00	$F = 5.02$
SD	465.45	282.55	351.11	$p < .01$
S. S. Income				
M	1457.00	1271.44	1070.33	$r = -.29$
SD	408.98	410.94	402.78	$p < .05$
% Over 50				
M	40.82	36.36	31.67	$r = -.30$
SD	8.13	9.84	8.92	$p < .01$
% < Ninth Grade				
M	10.53	13.47	13.44	$r = .25$
SD	3.66	4.81	2.92	$p < .05$
% Born in WI				
M	56.59_{ab}	72.44_a	78.11_b	$F = 13.67$
SD	14.44	11.19	7.64	$p < .0001$
% in Agriculture				
M	3.59_{ab}	9.36_a	11.78_b	$F = 5.45$
SD	3.24	7.51	9.35	$p < .01$
% in Construction				
M	10.35_a	7.14_a	6.89	$F = 3.92$
SD	5.48	3.56	2.93	$p < .05$

TABLE 2 (continued)

Variable	Amenity	NORC Bi-Focal	Convenience	
% in Transportation				
M	3.00_a	5.92_a	5.11	F = 4.20
SD	1.73	4.04	3.02	p < .05
% in Retail Sales				
M	22.12	18.25	18.78	r = − .23
SD	7.16	5.22	2.99	p < .05
% in Entertainment				
M	1.24	.69	.33	r = − .23
SD	1.86	1.04	1.00	p < .05

While these results are informative, they only distinguish particular characteristics of individual NORC types. Because it was our desire to offer an overall summary of the data as well as to provide a diagnostic tool for communities not included in our survey, we next performed a stepwise multiple discriminant analysis that maximized Rao's V. The goal was to identify variables that differentiate among the three NORC types. Because there were three types of NORCs, two discriminate functions were possible. However, only the first was statistically significant, producing a C^2 of 43.77 (p < .0001) and accounting for 98.05% of the total variance (canonical correlation = .72). The second function produced a nonsignificant C^2 of 1.24 and a canonical correlation of .15.

Four items significantly discriminated between the three types of NORCs. They were (a) the percentage of residents born in Wisconsin, (b) the percentage of employed persons working in transportation, (c) the percentage of employed persons working in retail sales, and (d) the percentage of residents over age 21 who received less than a ninth grade education (see Table 3).

The discriminant functions were successful in classifying 59.68% of the total cases. Specifically, 100% of Amenity NORCs, 36.1% of Bi-Focal NORCs, and 77.8% of Convenience NORCs were correctly classified (see Table 4).

TABLE 3. Variables Discriminating Between the Three Types of NORCs

Step	Variable	F to Enter	Change in V	Signif.
1	% Born in WI	13.67	27.34	$p < .001$
2	% in Transportation	6.75	19.25	$p < .001$
3	% in Retail Sales	2.76	10.01	$p < .01$
4	% < Ninth Grade	2.29	9.30	$p < .01$

TABLE 4. Percent of Cases Correctly Classified by NORC Type

Actual Group	# of Cases	Predicted Group Membership		
		1	2	3
Group 1	17	17	0	0
		(100.0%)	(0%)	(0%)
Group 2	36	5	13	18
		(13.9%)	(36.1%)	(50.0%)
Group 3	9	1	1	7
		(11.1%)	(11.1%)	(77.8%)

These results suggested that, while we could discriminate between Amenity and Convenience NORCs with some degree of accuracy, we were largely unable to determine Bi-Focal NORCs using Census data. To validate this interpretation further, we eliminated the Bi-Focal NORCs from the analysis and recomputed the discriminant analysis using only Amenity and Convenience NORCs. In this analysis, six of the 12 variables significantly differentiated between these two NORC types. These are shown in Table 5. Three of the four variables that discriminated among the three NORC types also discriminated between Amenity and Convenience NORCs (only the education variable dropped out). In addition, three other variables were significant. These were (a) the percentage of vacant housing, (b) per capita retirement income, and (c) the percentage of workers employed in the entertainment industry.

The discriminant function produced an eigenvalue of 5.19 (canoni-

TABLE 5. Variables Discriminating Between Amenity and Convenience NORCs

Step	Variable	F to Enter	Change in V	Signif.
1	% Born in WI	17.20	17.21	p < .001
2	% in Retail Sales	15.07	26.99	p < .001
3	% Vacant	5.75	17.83	p < .001
4	Per Capita Retirement Income	10.54	43.18	p < .001
5	% in Transportation	3.49	22.60	p < .001
6	% in Entertainment	1.47	11.73	p < .001

cal correlation = .92), and yielded a significant C^2 of 40.30 (p < .0001). Furthermore, the function successfully classified 100% of both Amenity and Convenience NORCs.

DISCUSSION

These results suggest that, while we can accurately discriminate between Amenity and Convenience NORCs using a relatively small group of Census variables, we cannot extend prediction to Bi-Focal NORCs. There are several potential explanations for this finding. First, it is possible that individuals who seek out Bi-Focal NORCs differ from other retirees on the basis of psychographic rather than demographic variables. As a result, relying solely on the demographic variables provided by the Census is an inaccurate method for classifying these residents. A second possibility is that the mismatch between our original sampling strategy (zip codes) and the level of the census data (cities, villages, and townships) was sufficient to make finer distinctions impossible. This mismatch could have proved troublesome in a number of ways. First, by including areas that were more that 50% covered by the zip code, we may have included individuals who were not in the original sample and exclude others who were. Furthermore, because zip codes in rural areas tend to cover large and diverse geographical areas, it is possible that multiple NORC types were contained within a single zip code. Thus, while the global NORC would be coded according to the dominant response pattern, smaller component communities with populations insufficient to influence the overall NORC designation may have been coded inaccurately. When these codes were compared to the more precise Census data, misfits would emerge.

Although discrimination of Bi-Focal NORCs was an insufficient base upon which to make policy recommendations, the clear distinction between Amenity and Convenience NORCs is none the less noteworthy. Communities featuring a high percentage of vacant housing (i.e., vacation homes), a comparatively high percentage of workers employed in entertainment, and high per capita retirement income are likely to continue to attract Amenity movers. In contrast, those communities with a high percentage of residents who were born in Wisconsin and a comparatively high percentage of workers employed in transportation and retail sales are likely destinations for Convenience movers. This information, while limited, already suggests some fruitful planning considerations. For example, Hunt et al. (1993) have shown that Amenity movers tend to remain in their homes, living independently, until it is no longer practicable for them to do so. At that point they move away from the area, often to be near children. Thus, while home-based health care would be attractive for Amenity movers, center-based health care would be likely to receive a much cooler reception. For Convenience movers, by comparison, center-based health care initiatives may prove much more profitable.

In summary, while Census data appear to provide adequate means for discriminating Amenity and Convenience NORCs, they are significantly less successful in classifying Bi-Focal NORCs. Further research is needed to determine whether this is the result of psychographic influences or if more refined sampling techniques would be successful in formulating a powerful diagnostic tool. Nonetheless, preliminary discrimination of Amenity and Convenience NORCs provides a powerful starting point for community planners.

REFERENCES

Bentley, Susan E. (1988). *Transfer payments in investment income in the nonmetro United States.* United States Department of Agriculture, Economic Research Service, Rural Development Research, Report No. 71.

Boehm, William T., and Pond, Martin T. (1976). Job location, retail purchasing patterns, and local economic development. *Growth and Change*, January, 7-12.

Briggs, R., and Rees, J. (1982). Control factors in the economic development of nonmetropolitan America. *Environment and Planning*, 14, 1645-1666.

Erikson, Rodney, and Huddleston, Jack. (1975). *Small community growth.* Madison, WI: Wisconsin State Planning Office.

Fagan, Mark. (1988). *Attracting retirees for economic development.* Jacksonville State University: Center for Economic Development and Business Research.

Fuguitt, Glenn V., and Bealle, Calvin L. (1993). The changing concentration of the older nonmetropolitan population, 1960-1990. *Journal of Gerontology,* 48(6), 5278-5288.

Fuguitt, Glenn V., and Tordella, Stephen J. (1980). Elderly net migration: The new trend of nonmetropolitan population change. *Research on Aging,* 2(2), 191-204.

Guhleman, Patricia, and Slesinger, Doris P. (1984). Wisconsin's elderly population, 1970-1980. *Population Notes,* Applied Population Laboratory, University of Wisconsin-Madison, No. 15.

Haas, William H., and Crandall, Lee A. (1988). Physician's views of retirement migrants' impact on rural medical practice. *Gerontologist,* 28(5), 663-666.

Harmston, Floyd K. (1979). *The study of the economic relationships of retired people in a small community.* Columbia, MO: Department of Agricultural Economics, University of Missouri.

Heaton, Tim B., Clifford, William B., and Fuguitt, Glenn V. (1981). Temporal shifts in the determinants of young and elderly migration in nonmetropolitan areas. *Social Forces,* 60(1), 41-60.

Hirschl, Thomas A., and Summers, Gene F. (1985). Shifts in rural income: The implications of unearned income for rural community development. *Research in Rural Sociology and Development,* 2, 127-141.

Hunt, Michael E., Marshall, Linda J., and Merrill, John L. (1993). The ABCs of rural naturally occurring retirement communities. Manuscript submitted for publication.

Li, Peter S., and MacLean, Brian D. (1989). Changes in the rural elderly population and their effects on the small town community: The case of Saskatchewan, 1971-1986. *Rural Sociology,* 54(2), 213-226.

Longino, Charles F., and Crown, William H. (1989). The migration of old money. *American Demographics,* 11(10), 28-31.

Richards, Bill. (1988). August 5. An influx of retirees pumps new vitality into distressed towns. *Wall Street Journal,* pp. 1, 6.

Siegal, Paul B., and Leuthold, Frank O. (1992). *Economic and fiscal impacts of Tellico Village, Loudon County, Tennessee.* Knoxville: University of Tennessee Agricultural Experimentation Station, Research Report 92-17.

Smith, Eldon D., Hackbart, Merlin M., and van Veen, Johannes. (1981). A modified regression base multiplier model. *Growth and Change,* 12, 17- 22.

Summers, Gene F., and Hirschl, Thomas A. (1985). Retirees as a growth industry. *USDA Rural Development Perspectives, 1984-1987.*

U.S. Bureau of Economic Analysis. (1986). Computer tape file supplied by Applied Population Laboratory, University of Wisconsin-Madison.

Voss, Paul, and Fuguitt, Glenn V. (1979). March. *Characteristics of recent migrants to Wisconsin's north country.* Paper presented at the meeting of the Population Interest Group, Madison, WI.

Wisconsin Department of Development. (1984). *Report 201.* Unpublished manuscript. Rural Housing Working Group, Madison, WI.

The Resident Services Coordinator Program: Bringing Service Coordination to Federally Assisted Senior Housing

Nancy W. Sheehan

SUMMARY. This article discusses a two-year federally funded on-site service coordination program, the Resident Services Coordinator Program, designed to increase elderly residents' ability to age in place in senior housing. The key component of the program is the placement of a Resident Services Coordinator, a social service professional, on-site in federally assisted senior housing. Evaluation of the program demonstrated the importance of on-site service coordination for both elderly residents and housing management. The implications of the program for shaping housing policy are presented. *[Article copies available for a fee from The Haworth Document Delivery Service: 1-800-342-9678. E-mail address: getinfo@haworthpressinc.com]*

Nancy W. Sheehan, PhD, is affiliated with the Travelers Center on Aging, University of Connecticut, Storrs, CT.

The author wishes to acknowledge the dedication and commitment of the key staff persons who were instrumental throughout every phase of the project: Ralph Cheyney, Chief of Social Services, CHFA, and Principal Investigator, Bette Myerson, Elderly Services Officer, CHFA, and Project Director, and Horace McCaulley, State of Connecticut, Elderly Services Division.

This project was supported in part by Award No. 90AM0439 from the Administration on Aging, Office of Human Development Services, Department of Health and Human Services, Washington, DC 20201. Grantees undertaking projects under government sponsorship are encouraged to express freely their findings and conclusions. Points of view or opinions do not, therefore, represent official Administration on Aging policy.

An earlier version of this paper was presented at the Annual Meeting of the Gerontological Society, New Orleans, LA (November 1993).

KEYWORDS. Aging in place senior housing, residence services, on-site resident services, implications for residents and management, housing policy

As elderly residents in senior housing age in place, increased public policy attention has focused on the development of supportive service models. These models seek to prolong the ability of frail elderly residents to remain living independently in senior housing and reduce the costs associated with unnecessary or premature nursing home placement. At present, approaches to service coordination in senior housing reflect several distinct approaches to addressing the needs of frail elderly residents. Three distinct approaches have been identified (Struyk et al., 1989). One approach involves deployment of a statewide service coordinator to assist housing managers in accessing community-based services. Under this approach, the statewide service coordinator provides training and technical assistance to housing managers to enable them to better serve the needs of elderly residents. The second approach involves the construction of congregate housing for elderly residents who require a more supportive environment than traditional senior housing provides. Under this approach, elderly residents who experience moderate to severe limitations in their ability to care for themselves are moved from independent senior housing to the more service-rich environment of congregate housing. No provisions are made for bringing services into independent senior housing. Finally, the third approach involves bringing services or service coordination into existing senior housing to meet the needs of elderly residents who are aging in place. Funds for services or service coordination may be provided by federal, state, or local housing sponsors.

Of these approaches to service coordination/delivery, the third approach has received the greatest attention from housing specialists, policy makers, and gerontologists. Under this approach, there are a wide variety of different models for bringing services into senior housing. In general, these different models share a similar goal of prolonging the ability of frail elderly to remain in independent senior housing and avoid unnecessary or premature nursing home placement. However, existing models of service coordination/delivery in senior housing have yet to be systematically evaluated to determine their effectiveness in meeting the elderly residents' needs.

This article discusses one model of service coordination in independent senior housing, the Resident Services Coordinator (RSC) Program. The RSC Program was initiated under a two-year demonstration grant from the Administration on Aging. The overall intent of the program was to bring service coordination into federally assisted senior housing by placing a Resident Services Coordinator on-site in the housing. The following discussion highlights the: (1) background of the program; (2) core components of the RSC program; (3) the evaluation of the program; and (4) policy implications of the RSC program.

BACKGROUND

Historically, the Connecticut Housing Finance Authority (CHFA) has been a leader and innovator in the area of elderly housing. In 1979, CHFA, recognizing the aging in place of residents, created the position of Social Services Coordinator to assist housing managers in meeting the needs of elderly residents. CHFA's commitment to meeting the needs of elderly residents was later expanded with the creation of a Social Services Unit within its Housing Management Division. Over time, as the numbers of functionally impaired elderly residents continued to grow, CHFA recognized the need to bring service coordination into senior housing to address elderly residents' needs.

With funding from the Administration on Aging, CHFA, working with the Connecticut Department on Aging (CDA) and Travelers Center on Aging, University of Connecticut (TCA), developed, implemented and evaluated the RSC Program. The RSC program was developed so that if it was successful it could be replicated in other senior housing complexes across the state and throughout the country.

RSC PROGRAM

The key component of the RSC Program is the deployment of a trained social service professional, a Resident Services Coordinator, on-site in senior housing. Hired as an employee of the management company, the RSC works with elderly and non-elderly disabled residents to ensure that they receive essential services to enable them to remain living independently in the community. The key functions performed by the RSC include: (1) identifying residents whose functional limitations place them "at risk;" (2) assessing the needs of each potentially "at risk" resident; (3) designing individualized strategies for working with residents experiencing some type of functional disability; (4) linking residents with services; (5) monitoring the delivery of services; (6) advocating for needed services; and (7) assisting with relocating frail elderly residents when necessary. RSCs work with on-site property managers to identify frail or "at risk" residents. In addition, other frail or "at risk" residents are identified through direct contacts with residents, family members, and community-based professionals. Each frail or "at risk" resident is evaluated to determine level of functional impairment, formal and informal services received and unmet service needs. For each frail or disabled resident, the RSC develops an individualized care plan and monitoring schedule. The RSC is also available to provide assistance to the more functionally independent residents.

In addition to these primary functions, the RSC also functions to: (1) educate residents about their rights, entitlements, etc.; (2) educate housing management and staff about aging and aging services; and (3) promote a positive social climate in the housing complex that enhances residents' psychosocial well-being. (A detailed description of the components of the RSC Program is presented in the project's Operational Manual, *The Elderly Supportive Services Program: Bringing Service Coordination into Senior Housing,* Sheehan, 1992.)

DEMONSTRATION PHASE

As a two-year model project, the demonstration phase involved the design, implementation, and evaluation of the program. Three private housing management companies participated in the program. Each management company designated two sites to participate in the program. Only sites that had an on-site property manager and had been in operation at least six years were eligible. Each company agreed to pay 1/4 of the full-time RSC salary during Year I, 3/4 of the salary during Year II, and create a permanent RSC position, if the program proved successful. During the first year, each RSC worked in a single housing complex. During Year II, each assumed responsibility for an additional senior housing complex. Consequently, a total of six complexes participated in the demonstration phase. Five of the six housing sites were relatively large (110+ units), ranging in size from 113 to 155 units. The remaining senior housing site was small, consisting of only 38 units.

The characteristics of the elderly residents living in the demonstration sites indicated the typical resident was white, female, and living alone. Although there was some variability in resident characteristics across the six complexes, the most common demographic profile of elderly residents indicated that a significant proportion experienced impairments in their ability to carry out essential activities of daily living. Table 1 presents the demographic profiles of elderly residents living in the Year I, Year II sites, and small random samples of elderly

TABLE 1. Demographic Characteristics of Elderly Residents in the Demonstration and Comparison Sites

	Demonstration Sites		Comparison Sites	
	Year I	Year II	Comp 1	Comp 2
Age	76 yrs	73.4 yrs	78 yrs	74 yrs
Gender				
Female	80%	81%	85%	69%
Male	20%	19%	15%	31%
Marital Status				
Married	21%	15%	8%	23%
Widowed	56%	57%	54%	23%
Div/Sep	14%	17%	15%	46%
Single	9%	11%	23%	8%
Race				
White	93%	89%	100%	100%
African-Am	5%	9%		
Hispanic	2%	2%		
Av. Tenancy	6 yrs	5.1 yrs	8.6 yrs	5.6 yrs
Health				
Fair/Poor	51%	53%	31%	39%
ADL*	38%	22%	31%	39%
IADL*	93%	57%	77%	92%

*Difficulty with at least one activity

residents living in two senior housing sites not participating in the program. Since differences exist between residents in the demonstration sites and comparison sites, any comparisons between the two can only be suggestive. However, for all sites, small, but substantial numbers of elderly residents experience limitations in their ability to carry out the basic activities of daily living.

EVALUATION OF RSC PROGRAM

The evaluation design employed: (1) key informant interviews with on-site property managers, RSCs, and management company representatives; (2) case studies of elderly residents at risk of nursing home placement; (3) weekly activity logs completed by RSCs; (4) pretest-posttest interviews with elderly residents in the demonstration sites and random samples of residents living in two other senior housing sites. An overview of the findings from the key informant interviews and pretest-posttest interviews is summarized below. A complete report of the project's findings is contained in the Final Report (Sheehan, 1993).

Key Informant Interviews. Interviews explored experiences in implementing the program, interpersonal relationships and tensions among the key actors involved (residents, sites managers, and management representatives), experiences in enacting the RSC role, circumstances surrounding relocation when a frail resident could no longer remain in the housing, and perceptions of both the advantages and disadvantages of the program. Each interview was tape recorded and later transcribed. Open-ended responses were analyzed to identify the major themes associated with the program. Based upon these interviews, a number of broad based themes emerged. In some cases, these themes were initially associated with problems or conflicts that were later resolved. Most were associated with the negotiation of expectations, roles, and relationships as the RSC role was introduced into the housing. Critical themes or issues that emerged for housing managers were their shared concerns about giving up aspects of their previous role and ambiguity concerning the exact nature of the role of the RSC. The intensity of these concerns ranged from a general uneasiness about how their role was changing in response to the presence of the RSC to strong resentment about the presence of the RSC. Over time, most on-site property managers accepted the presence of the RSC. For these on-site property managers, the RSC was viewed as a valuable resource enabling them to direct more time and attention to their management functions. Only one housing manager never acknowledged the value of the RSC in easing her management responsibilities. This manager, who strongly valued the social service aspects of her role, felt she was totally capable of meeting the needs of all elderly residents.

Ambiguity concerning the exact nature of the RSC role was shared by both housing managers and RSCs. Although the functions of the RSC role were identified, both managers and RSCs expressed confusion concerning the specific allocation of time among these multiple activities and functions. Several housing managers expressed their desire that the RSC should serve as an Activities Director. Over time, the respective concerns of the RSCs and on-site property managers were resolved. Initially, RSCs expected that a major portion of their time would be spent linking residents with services; experience in the role, however, revealed that in reality they spent much less time arranging services. The words of one RSC capture the changing view of the role of Resident Services Coordinator: "Now, I don't think it's that elemental [linking residents up with services]. It's much broader and gets into a lot more trying to get at what's behind the stated purpose in coming to see me." Another RSC noted: "I mean if somebody needs a homemaker, it doesn't take a skilled person to pick up the phone and call a homemaking company, but it takes a good deal of skill . . . for a person to spend ten visits building the trust level . . . so the person might consider getting a homemaker."

For RSCs, confidentiality and supervision emerged as critical concerns. An ongoing tension between RSCs and property managers involved confidentiality of the information that elderly residents shared with the RSC and the on-site property managers' desire to be informed about residents' needs and changing circumstances. Since the success of the RSC's efforts depends on her/his ability to assure residents that the information that they share is confidential, the RSC must be able to ensure confidentiality. However, the on-site property manager expects to be informed about the RSC's activities and the changing circumstances of residents being assisted. RSCs generally resolved this tension by sharing very general information with the on-site property manager that did not jeopardize the confidential nature of the relationship.

A second concern that emerged from the perspective of the RSCs was the need for ongoing supervision. Given the nature of their work, RSCs expressed the desire for access to ongoing case conferences and supervision. Within the housing management companies, none of the RSCs' supervisors had the necessary background or training to provide such supervision.

The final concern that emerged involved the negotiation of an effective working relationship between the RSC and on-site property manager. The ability to establish a positive working relationship was related to mutual professional respect and understanding of the value and respective functions that the RSC and on-site manager performed to benefit elderly residents. Significant tensions were revealed between a RSC and housing manager when the housing manager expressed frustration with the RSC's activities. According to this housing manager, she could not understand why it took the RSC *so long* to arrange services for residents. According to this on-site housing manager, she could solve any problem that residents brought to her with a single phone call.

Finally, key informant interviews identified numerous benefits associated with the program. Housing management personnel noted that the program: improved the quality of life for residents; reduced the risk of nursing home placement; enhanced the building's reputation; and achieved financial savings for the management company. Savings were linked to lower turnover and vacancy rates and improved upkeep and maintenance of units. From the view of on-site property managers, RSC's freed them from the responsibility to care for the support needs of elderly residents and allowed them to concentrate on the management functions of their job. In addition to providing a resource to deal with the day-to-day support needs of frail elderly residents, the presence of the RSC offered management a strategy for more effectively dealing with lease non-compliance issues. More specifically, using a "good cop/bad cop" strategy, the manager's effectiveness in dealing with problem situations is enhanced. In situations involving lease non-compliance, the housing manager confronts the resident with the unacceptability of the situation ("bad cop") and then suggests that the RSC ("good cop") is available to assist the resident in addressing the lease compliance problem. The RSC confirms that the problem exists and helps the resident understand how the situation is placing his/her tenancy in jeopardy.

While management generally viewed the program as resulting in improved management efficiency, RSCs focused on the program's benefits to residents. RSCs noted that the program offers residents a personal level of contact ("a much more human level of contact") for monitoring and supporting frail elderly residents. They also noted that the flexibility of the program enables RSCs to address both the individual and aggregate needs of residents in a particular complex.

Pretest-Posttest Interviews with Elderly Residents. Interviews were conducted with elderly residents living in six senior housing demonstration sites and two comparison sites. Response rates for the Year I and Year II sites were 72 percent (N = 203) and 81 percent (N = 277), respectively. For the two comparison sites, the response rate was 81 percent (N = 26). Separate analyses were conducted for the Year I, Year II, and comparison sites. Since the comparison sites were not matched to the demonstration sites, any comparisons between the demonstration and comparison sites can only be somewhat suggestive of possible time-related changes occurring.

Pretest interviews were conducted in each complex prior to the program's initiation. Posttest interviews were conducted approximately eight months after implementation in each complex. The interview assessed: (1) residents' interest and willingness to participate in the program; (2) perceived benefits of the RSC program; and (3) health and functional ability, unmet needs, utilization of formal services, housing satisfaction, frequency of social interaction in the complex, and psychosocial well-being.

The majority of elderly residents expressed an interest in learning more about the program and an openness to the possibility of using the program. Eight months after the program began, the overwhelming majority of elderly residents agreed that residents had benefited from the program. Analyses of open-ended responses from Year I residents attributed numerous benefits to the RSC program. These included: emotional support; immediate help when problems arise; peace of mind/security; information and referral; and help for frail elderly residents. In two of the three Year I sites, the most frequently cited benefit was the provision of emotional support ("someone to talk to," "a shoulder to cry on," etc.), while residents at the third site most frequently valued the importance of available assistance when needed ("when help is needed it's available"). Other benefits were: a sense of security/peace of mind (e.g., "security knowing that should you need assistance, she's there to act as a resource," "helps with a feeling of well-being," etc.); information and referral (e.g., "someone to ask questions to," "information when you need it," "someone to link you up with services if you don't know how to get them"); and socialization (e.g., "helps bring people out of their apartments").

Some residents primarily focused on the benefits to frail residents. These residents noted the importance of the RSC for: "the needs of people who aren't mobile," "others who have heart problems, shut-ins," etc. Only six elderly residents reported either dissatisfaction or no perceived benefits from the program and two indicated that they were unaware of the program. These residents generally indicated that if they had a problem they would go to the housing manager. In contrast, residents who valued the program generally noted that management was too busy to handle many of the problems that elderly residents experience.

A series of dependent t-tests examined significant changes in health, functional ability, housing satisfaction, social involvement, and psychosocial well-being. Separate t-tests were computed for the Year I, Year II and comparison samples to explore possible changes over time. Additional analyses compared changes for frail and non-frail elderly subsamples drawn exclusively from the demonstration sites. Over time, most health indicators evidenced significant declines. However, comparative health (perceived health in comparison to age peers) of frail residents showed significant improvement for both the Year I ($t = 3.0$, $df = 56$, $p < .004$) and Year II ($t = 3.5$, $df = 34$, $p < 001$) sites. Further, Year I and Year II frail residents evidenced significant improvements in functional ability. More specifically, frail residents in Year I sites evidenced improved ADL ($t = 4.6$, $df = 59$, $p < .0001$) and IADL ($t = 4.3$, $df = 59$, $p < .0001$) functioning. A similar pattern of improved ADL ($t = 5.1$, $df = 36$, $p < .0001$) and IADL ($t = 6.4$, $df = 36$, $p < .0001$) functioning for frail residents was noted for the Year II sites. No such positive changes were noted for either the comparison group or non-frail elderly residents in the demonstration sites. In fact, non-frail elderly in Year I and Year II sites showed significant declines in ADL and IADL performance, while the comparison group showed no significant change.

Housing satisfaction increased significantly for both frail and non-frail elderly residents in Year I and Year II sites (Year I frail, $t = -3.6$, $df = 57$, $p < .006$; Year I non-frail, $t = -3.8$, $df = 96$, $p < .0003$); (Year II frail, $t = -3.5$, $df = 43$, $p < .001$; Year II non-frail, $t = -7.3$, $df = 209$, $p < .0001$). Increased levels of social participation in the complex were also noted for both frail (Year I, t = 3.9, *df* = 50, p < .0003 and Year II, t = 3.9, *df* = 30, p < .0005) and non-frail (Year I, t = 3.0, *df* = 84, p < .004 and Year II, t = 6.7, *df* = 131, p < .0001). For residents living in the comparison sites, a slight increase was noted in frequency of social activity at one site and no change at the second. Finally, positive changes in life satisfaction (t = − 3.0, *df* = 58, p < .004) and overall affect (t = − 2.3, *df* = 58, p < .03) were noted for frail residents in Year I sites. Decreased negative affect was also noted for frail (t = 2.3, *df* = 58, p < .02) and non-frail (t = 2.2, *df* = 93, p < .03) for the Year I sites. No significant changes were noted in life satisfaction for Year II site residents or the comparison groups. For the Year II sites, the only significant change was a decrease in positive affect among non-frail residents (t = 2.5, *df* = 97, p < .01).

SIGNIFICANCE OF THE RESULTS

From the perspective of housing management, on-site property managers, RSCs, and elderly residents, there is a general consensus concerning the success of the program. For management, the program eases the burden on on-site managers, improves the quality of life of residents, and results in financial savings. Overall, the RSC serves as a resource to management to more effectively address the problems that arise as elderly residents age in place. The commitment of all three management companies to make the RSC position a permanent, full-time position is convincing evidence of the programs' success. From a cost-benefit perspective, the costs of hiring a trained social service professional to work with elderly and non-elderly residents are outweighed by the rewards (benefits) derived from the program. On-site property managers noted that the presence of the RSC frees them to devote more of their time to management functions. Elderly residents also endorsed the benefits derived from the program: availability of assistance in times of need; emotional support; information and referral; and security. The words of one elderly resident underscore the importance of the RSC in her life, " I would be lost without her." Other residents valued the availability of the RSC in the event that they might become ill or need assistance. The availability of RSCs to respond to the assistance needs of *all* residents is an essential component of the program. Given the complex, dynamic changes that occur among the elderly, a sizable proportion of functionally independent residents anticipate that their needs for assistance will increase in the near future (McGory et al., 1992).

The positive impact of the program on residents' housing satisfaction, frequency of social participation, and functional ability provides an optimistic view of how increasing the supportive nature of the environment can increase residents' competencies (Lawton, 1983).

LIMITATIONS

Although the evaluation of the RSC Program generally indicates the positive impact of the program on frail elderly residents' competencies (health, functional ability, social participation, and psychosocial well-being) (Lawton, 1983), there are several limitations that must be acknowledged in the evaluation design that limit generalizations regarding the program's impact. First, possible bias in the responses of key informants must be acknowledged. Key informants may have been inclined to present an overly positive view of the program's benefit. Further, some elderly residents may have been reluctant to criticize the program. If such bias exists, then the results must be interpreted with some caution. However, it is important to point out that a small number of respondents did express negative responses about aspects of the program. Second, the inability to match residents from the demonstration sites and comparison sites limits the conclusions that can be drawn concerning the impact of the program. These results must, therefore, be interpreted with some caution. A third problem that affects the interpretation of the results is that almost 1/3 of residents assisted by the RSC did not participate in the initial interview. Finally, the limited amount of time between the pretest and posttest interviews represents a significant problem. Longer term follow-up interviews would inevitably influence the nature of the findings. Overall, despite these acknowledged limitations, there is evidence that the program had a positive impact on elderly residents.

POLICY IMPLICATIONS OF THE PROJECT

The Resident Services Coordinator Program offers policy makers a viable model of service coordination in federally assisted senior housing designed to enable frail elderly residents to remain living independently in the community. While other supportive service models in senior housing exist, such as the Robert Wood Johnson Supportive Services Program in Senior Housing (SSPSH) and the Congregate Housing Services Program (CHSP), there are several advantages associated with the RSC Program that should be considered. First, the program works individually with frail elderly residents to determine their service needs and links needy residents with essential services to optimize their independence. Rather than the service brokering approach of the SSPSH which identifies a package of supportive services that the majority of residents are willing to pay for, the RSC Program focuses on individual residents' needs. Since many frail elderly residents may be reluctant to express their need for services, the efforts of the RSC are geared toward helping elderly residents to identify their needs.

Second, the RSC Program is more flexible in addressing the needs of all residents than the Congregate Housing Services Program. The CHSP requires eligible program participants to need assistance with at least three ADL activities (eating, dressing, bathing, grooming, getting in and out of bed, household management activities). Under the RSC Program, assistance is available to both frail and non-frail elderly residents. Programs that restrict eligibility to only frail elderly residents, such as the CHSP, potentially stigmatize elderly program participants and may prevent eligible residents from applying for the program. Anecdotal remarks from several former elderly residents who participated in a CHSP program underscore some of the negative feelings associated with a program for frail elderly residents. In the words of one former CHSP program participant, "I'd rather be dead than have to go back on the program." While this attitude cannot be said to reflect those of the majority of CHSP participants, there may be a substantial number of elderly residents whose independence and self-esteem is threatened by involvement in a program for "frail elderly" residents.

A third advantage of the RSC Program is the fact that the RSC is hired as an employee of the management company. Policy initiatives to encourage management companies to hire a Resident Services Coordinator should be explored. If management companies perceive the program to be cost effective and beneficial to both management and residents, they are likely to initiate the program. Based upon their experiences with the program, all the management companies involved in the demonstration program committed resources to make the RSC position a full-time, permanent position in their company.

Another advantage of the RSC program is its recognition of the importance of creating a positive social climate in which residents can thrive. Programs that exclusively focus on addressing the functional limitations of frail elderly residents fail to address the potential for frail or disabled residents to continue to grow. Knowledge and understanding of the social dynamics in senior housing are essential for creating an environment that promotes feelings of usefulness and well-being. As part of the RSC role, service coordinators are expected to reach out to socially isolated residents to encourage their involvement and participation. The importance of addressing the psychosocial needs of residents is underscored by earlier longitudinal research that indicated that over time elderly residents experience gradual, progressive reductions in their social space and social involvement. Supportive service programs must, therefore, be flexible enough to address the needs of the whole person.

While few question the value of "service coordination" programs in senior housing, a critical examination of existing models is needed to determine how each operates in senior housing. Issues that need to be addressed include: "To what extent do 'consumer-driven models' focusing on service brokering meet the comprehensive support needs of severely impaired elderly residents?" and "To what extent do models that restrict services to frail elderly residents create an unnecessary stigma for residents receiving services?"

As private housing management companies struggle to meet the needs of their aging residents, they should consider the RSC program as a successful, replicable model for responding to the aging in place of residents. From the perspective of the federal government, the program offers a cost-effective approach for ensuring that the needs of aging residents will be met. Consequently, the federal government and state housing finance agencies should explore financial incentives to encourage private management companies to implement the RSC program in federally assisted housing.

REFERENCES

Lawton, M.P. (1983). Environment and other determinants of well-being in older persons. *The Gerontologist, 23,* 349-357.

McGory, W.C., McFarland, A.S. & Kingson, E. (November 1992). Social service needs of elders in Boston Public Housing. Paper presented at the Annual Meeting of the Gerontological Society of America, Washington, DC.

Sheehan, N.W. (1992). The Elderly Supportive Services Program: Bringing service coordination into senior housing. Storrs, CT: University of Connecticut.

Sheehan, N.W. (1993). The Elderly Supportive Services Programs' Resident Services Coordinator Model. Final Report (Award No. 90AM0439) submitted to the Administration on Aging, U.S. Department of Health and Human Services, Washington, DC.

Struyk, R.J., Page, D.P., Newman, S., Carroll, M., Cohen, B. & Wright, P. (1989). Providing supportive services to the frail elderly in federally assisted housing. Washington, DC: The Urban Institute Press.

Social Support and Depression Among Low Income Elderly

William Lee Bothell
Joel Fischer
Cullen Hayashida

SUMMARY. Demographic, functional and social characteristics of residents living in a low-income senior housing complex are explored. These variables and perceptions of social support were analyzed for their effects on depression. The strongest predictor of depression was perceptions of social support. The findings are consistent with the research which shows that support through family and friends is important to consider when older adults experience health problems that lead to functional disability. *[Article copies available for a fee from The Haworth Document Delivery Service: 1-800-342-9678. E-mail address: getinfo@haworth pressinc.com]*

KEYWORDS. Low income senior housing, depression, social supports, characteristics of low-income residents, functional disability

Numerous studies have been conducted on the elderly in senior housing throughout the U.S. (David, Moos, & Kahn 1981; Lemke & Moos 1986; Macken, 1986). To date, however, few have reviewed the status of elderly residents and their informal caregivers while they are residing in senior housing units. Given the major changes taking place

---

William Lee Bothell, Joel Fischer, and Cullen Hayashida are all affiliated with the University of Hawai'i School of Social Work.

[Haworth co-indexing entry note]: "Social Support and Depression Among Low Income Elderly." Bothell, William Lee, Joel Fischer, and Cullen Hayashida. Co-published simultaneously in *Journal of Housing for the Elderly* (The Haworth Press, Inc.) Vol. 13, No. 1/2, 1999, pp. 51-63; and: *Making Aging in Place Work* (ed: Leon A. Pastalan) The Haworth Press, Inc., 1999, pp. 51-63. Single or multiple copies of this article are available for a fee from The Haworth Document Delivery Service [1-800-342-9678, 9:00 a.m. - 5:00 p.m. (EST). E-mail address: getinfo@haworthpressinc.com].

in federal and state reimbursements for seniors in nursing homes, it is anticipated that the nursing home bed supply will remain limited for the foreseeable future. Therefore, an understanding of the physical and mental health of elderly residents along with their social support networks will be critical in preventing or postponing premature long-term care nursing home placements.

LITERATURE REVIEW

Previous Research

The role played by social support in predicting institutionalization of the elderly has generated considerable research. Much of this work centers on investigations of the direct effect of social support on institutional risk without considering other factors that might affect that risk. For example, older people are less likely to be institutionalized who are currently married (Brody, Poulshock, & Masciocchi, 1978; Cohen, Tell, & Wallack, 1986; Dunlop, 1973; Greenberg & Ginn, 1979; Hughes, Manheim, Edelman, & Conrad, 1987; McCoy & Edwards, 1981; Palmore, 1976; Shapiro & Tate, 1988; Vicente, Wiley, & Carrington, 1979; Weissert & Cready, 1989); who have children in the home or nearby (Brody, Poulshock, & Masciocchi, 1978; Morris, Sherwood, & Gutkin, 1988; Wan & Weissert, 1981); or who have relatives or friends willing to provide the necessary care (Brock & O'Sullivan, 1985; Greenberg & Ginn, 1979; McAuley & Prohaska, 1982; Smallegan, 1985; Smyer, 1980).

Research shows that most elderly individuals have contact with others. Lowenthal and Haven (1968) referred to isolates as those having only casual contacts or no contacts with others for a two-week period prior to the interview. Peters and Kaiser (1985) report that most have friends and neighbors well into later life, few are isolated, and only about one in five have no confidants. Chappell (1987) reports that sixteen percent of elderly persons have no confidants and only four percent have no companion. Companions are friends who people see on a regular basis; they interact on a social level but do not get too personal with each other. Confidants, on the other hand, are friends who share personal problems with each other and do not hesitate to ask each other for help if needed (Peters and Kaiser, 1985).

Relevant Conceptualization

Support through family and friends is important to consider when older adults experience health problems which lead to functional disability, because they frequently turn to those in their social support networks for assistance with their activities of daily living (Krause, 1990). Evidence is accumulating that social support, particularly from patients' families, can affect compliance with medical regimens and hasten recovery from illness (Becker and Maiman, 1980).

In addition to the family, other sources of emotional support such as close friendships have been shown to act as buffers against stress and enhancers of personal health (Cassell, 1976). Pursuing the idea of social support as a buffer against the adverse effects of illness and loss, Maquire (1980) discussed the potential of human networks to assist individuals to cope with transition, stress, physical problems and social emotional problems without having to resort to the still somewhat stigmatized formal social services.

Along with social support from family and friends functional disability is an especially relevant stressor to include in a study of older adults because it is frequently encountered in later life (Arling, 1987; Kahn, Wetherington, & Ingersoll-Dayton, 1990; Ulbrich & Warheit, 1989).

Purpose of Study

This study is an exploratory investigation of a low-income senior housing facility in Honolulu that will examine factors affecting depression in elderly residents. The information was collected from October 1990 to March 1993 in semi-structured interviews. The study itself will first report on the social/demographic characteristics of the residents. Informal social support through family caregivers, friends, and participation in any outside group activity will be identified through an interview schedule developed by the researchers.

The Provision of Social Relations (PSR; Turner et al., 1983) instrument was used to measure the respondent's satisfaction with social support through family and friends.

Finally, depression was measured using the Generalized Contentment Scale (GCS; Hudson, 1982) comparing those residents who are socially isolated as opposed to those who have social support networks operating in their lives.

This study is an attempt to isolate variables that predict depression in the elderly living in a low income housing project. The significance of this study lies in attempting to isolate variables that can be of importance to those planning and working with the elderly in order to combat and prevent depression.

Hypothesis

Greater informal social support networks from family, friends, and outside activities as identified from the interview schedule and measured with the Provision of Social Relations (PSR) instrument leads to less depression for elderly residents, as measured by the Generalized Contentment Scale (GCS).

METHOD

Subjects

The initial 135 subjects of this study were all residents in a low income housing project for the elderly in Honolulu, Hawai'i managed by the Hawai'i Housing Authority. The residents varied in age from 40 to 91 years with a mean age of 74.93 (SD = 9.62). Most of the residents, 92 (68.1%), are women and single. In reviewing the marital status of the residents further, only 18 (13.3%) have never married, 54 (40%) are widowed and 35 (25.9%) have been divorced or separated. Only 28 (20.7%) were married at the time of this study.

Ethnically, the residents were characteristic of the multi-ethnic nature of Hawaii's aging population. Japanese and Japanese Americans were the largest group with 53 (39.3%). There were 24 Chinese subjects (17.8%), 15 Caucasians (11.1%), and the remaining 43 (31.8%) were compromised of Koreans, Filipinos, Hawaiians or part-Hawaiians, Portuguese, Puerto Ricans, and Samoans.

The average length of stay was 8.3 years (SD = 6.2). Residents varied in length of residence from eight months to 21.6 years. There was a relatively large number of recent residents (25.7%) within the past three years while the remaining residents were roughly equally distributed along the length of stay continuum from 4 to 21 years.

The residents were divided into four groups of informal social support in preliminary interviews based on self-reports of contacts with family, friends, and outside activities (such as church activities). Group One (n = 20) had no support. Group Two (n = 24) had support through one of the three identified supports. Group Three (n = 56) had two types of support, and Group Four (n=32) identified all three of the supports.

All of the residents in Group One were followed up in a second interview to administer the Provision of Social Relations (PSR) instrument and the Generalized Contentment Scale (GCS). Of the 20 residents who were approached, 15 (75%) interviews were completed; three residents refused and two said they were feeling too sick to fill out the instruments. A random sample of 15 was selected from Group Four (n = 32) in order to compare the results of the PSR and GCS in the two groups that reported the two extremes of social support (none versus all three sources of support).

Materials

The quantitative interview information for the first interview was obtained using an interview schedule that was developed by the researchers. The schedule was divided into three sections: (1) Socio-demographic information; (2) Health status indicators based on Activities of Daily Living (ADL) and Instrumental Activities of Daily Living (IADL) scores; and (3) measures of social support through family, friends, and outside activities.

Social support was measured by the amount of good friends (companions) and the amount of reliable friends (confidants) the residents had within the housing project along with the amount of family support. Indications of life satisfaction were measured using the residents' sense of perceived loneliness, amount of group activities and their general satisfaction with the frequency of visits from their family.

The interviews required between twenty minutes and one hour to conduct. Of the 135 tenants who were approached, 129 were successfully interviewed for a response rate of 95 percent. Interpreters were required for the few Korean, Japanese, Filipino, and Chinese speaking tenants within the facility. There were six residents who could not be contacted. No one actually refused to be interviewed.

The activities of Daily Living Scale (ADL) was developed by Katz and his colleagues and has been used to measure physical and functional disability for several years (Katz, Ford, Moskowitz, Jackson, & Jaffee, 1963; Katz, Hedrick, & Henderson, 1979). The interview schedule included the ADL scale which focuses on quite specific and basic functional activities: bathing, dressing, toileting, transferring, eating, walking, and grooming. Ratings are made by both patient and observer. The temporal dimension of the scale is limited to the present, which includes the two-week period prior to the evaluation. Actual performance, rather than potential capabilities, is measured, so that motivation and interest levels play a key role in the assessment outcomes. Items are rated on a 3-point scale, with each item yielding an independence/dependence score (Hickey, 1980). The ADL has been shown to be reliable through simultaneous observations that showed differences in less than 1 of 20 evaluations. Scores have been correlated with mobility and house confinement after discharge from the hospital (Kane & Kane, 1984).

The Instrumental Activities of Daily Living (IADL) scale includes a range of activities more complex than those needed for personal care (Katz et al., 1979). The IADL score focuses on more difficult daily tasks of living: shopping, meal preparation, light housekeeping, medication management, financial management, telephone use and mobility outside the home. These items are also rated on a 3-point scale, with each item yielding an independence-dependence score. The IADL has a reproducibility coefficient of .94 (Kane & Kane, 1984).

The second set of interviews included administration of the PSR and GCS. The Provision of Social Relations (PSR) is a 15-item instrument designed to measure components of social support. The PSR is one of the few instruments that examines the environmental variable of social support (or, at least, the respondent's perceptions). The PSR has good internal consistency, with alphas that range from .75 to .87. It also has good concurrent validity correlating significantly with the Kaplan Scale of Social Support. The PSR is negatively correlated with several measures of psychological distress, indicating that the PSR is not confounded by item content measuring psychological distress (Corcoran & Fischer, 1987). Higher scores on the PSR indicate lower perceived support.

The Generalized Contentment Scale (GCS) is a 25-item scale that is designed to measure the degree, severity, or magnitude of nonpsychotic depression. A particular advantage of the GCS is a cutting score of 30 (plus or minus 5), with scores above 30 indicating that the respondent has a clinically significant problem and scores below 30 indicating the individual has no such problem. The GCS has a mean alpha of .92, indicating excellent internal consistency, and an excellent (low) S.E.M. of 4.56. The GCS also has excellent stability with a two hour test-retest correlation of .94. The GCS has good concurrent validity, correlating .85 and .76 with the Beck Depression Inventory and .92 and .81 for two samples using the Zung Depression Inventory. The GCS has excellent known-groups validity, discriminating significantly between members of a group judged to be clinically depressed and those judged not to be depressed. The GCS also has good construct validity, correlating poorly with a number of measures with which it should not correlate, and correlating at high levels with several measures with which it should, such as self-esteem, happiness, and sense of identity (Corcoran & Fischer, 1987). Higher scores on the GCS indicate greater depression.

Procedure

The participant observation data were made possible through the assignment of one of the researchers as a student intern at the housing facility. In that capacity, the student intern provided services such as security, emergency referrals, fostering resident activities and fielding maintenance requests particularly after normal working hours. Acting in this official capacity, it was possible to conduct participant observations and home visits while remaining on site over the course of three years. From this vantage point, it was possible to develop a fuller understanding of the personality of each resident and gain their trust and rapport.

The interview schedule was used to identify the levels of informal social support and functional status of the residents. As identified through the interview schedule, the PSR and GCS instruments were administered in follow-up interviews with isolated and supported residents. Isolated residents had no support through family, friends, and outside activities and supported residents had support through all three.

In addition to the above, this study also obtained part of the data from the housing authority's files on the residents. All of the demographic data on the first page of the interview schedule were obtained in this manner. This assured the study would have valid information on marital status, sex, ethnicity, date of birth or age, and date of occupancy or length of stay. Obtaining this information from the housing authority's files also minimized the need to embarrass the resident with personal questions. Because demographic information was collected in this manner, it was possible to obtain information on all 135 residents or 100 percent of the cases.

The researchers identified supported as opposed to non-supported residents through the interview schedule. Twenty residents did not have social support through family, friends and outside activities and 32 residents had social support through all three. All 20 of the non-supported residents were approached to complete the PSR and GCS instruments. Three refused and two said that they were too ill to be bothered, producing a completion rate of 75%. A random sample of 15 residents was selected from the supported residents to compare the two groups on the effects of social support on depression.

RESULTS

The mean age of the 30 residents who were identified as supported versus isolated was 74.1 (SD = 11.56). Residents who were supported had a mean age of 78.3 (SD = 8.5). Residents who were not supported had a mean age of 71.4 (SD = 11.3). The difference between these scores was statistically significant (t = -2.33, p < .05).

Most of the respondents 21 (70%), were women. In reviewing the marital status of the sample, it was found that only 7 (23.3%) had never married, 11 (36.7%) were widowed and 8 (26.7%) had been divorced of separated. Only 4 (13.3%) currently were married.

Regarding ethnicity, there were 15 (50%) Japanese respondents, 5 (16.7%) Chinese, 3 (10%) Caucasians, and the remaining 7 (23.3%) were Korean, Filipino, Hawaiian or part-Hawaiian, Puerto Rican, Samoan or other groups.

The mean length of stay was 96.87 (SD = 74.04) months. Residents who were supported had a longer length of stay at 129.36 (SD = 87) months than residents who were not supported 68.04 (SD = 39.72). The difference between the two groups was statistically significant (t = -3.46, p < .001).

The mean ADL score for the entire sample was 13.8 (SD = .805). Residents who were supported had a mean ADL score of 13.1 (SD = 1.7). Residents who were not supported had a mean ADL score of 14 (completely independent). The difference between these two scores was statistically significant (t = no variance in support group, p < .001).

The mean IADL score for the entire sample was 13.6 (SD = .669). Residents who were supported had a mean IADL score of 12.7 (SD = 1.89). Residents who were not supported had a mean IADL score of 13.8 (SD .55). The difference between these two groups was statistically significant (t = 2.90, p < .01).

The mean PSR score for the entire sample was 43.5 (SD = 15.2). For the support group, the mean PSR score was 31.4 (SD = 10.9), and for the non-supported group, the mean was 55.6 (SD = 10.9). The difference between these two scores was statistically significant (t = 7.29, p < .001).

The mean GCS score for the entire sample was 46.2 (SD = 14.8), considerably above the cutting score of 30, indicating that on the whole, this group was moderately depressed. The mean GCS score for the supported group was 36.3 (SD = 10.7), and for the non-supported group was 56.07 (SD = 11.5), well above the clinical cutting point of 30 (plus or minus 5). The difference between the groups was statistically significant (t = 4.85, p < .001).

Preliminary regression diagnostics revealed that the data were appropriate for a multiple regression equation (no outliers, data normally distributed). Group membership (supported versus non-supported), as expected, was highly correlated with PSR scores (− .809) and was the only significant predictor of PSR (t = − 3.645, p < .01). Therefore, because of the problem of multicollinearity, group membership was dropped from the equation.

The rest of the data were entered into a multiple regression equation as follows: (1) length of stay, (2) sex (dummy coded), (3) marital status (dummy coded), (4) IADL Total score, (5) ethnicity (dummy coded into four categories), (6) PSR score, (7) age, and (8) ADL Total score. The results of the multiple regression of these variables on GCS scores are displayed in Table 1.

As can be seen from the data in Table 1, the overall regression equation was significant. The beta weights showed that the PSR contributed the most to explaining depression among the elderly in this sample, followed by length of stay in the housing project, and the scores on the IADL. Of these, only the PSR was statistically significant.

The R square for the multiple regression equation showed that the predictor variables explained almost 78% of the variance in depression scores. However, the adjusted R square, due to the size of the

TABLE 1. Multiple Regression with GCS as Criterion Variable

Variable	B	SE B	Beta	T	Sig T
STAY	−.04560	.03040	−.22733	−1.500	.1485
SEX	.11609	4.01442	.03747	.029	.9772
MARISTAT	−1.43227	1.75141	−.09453	−.818	.4227
IADLTOT	−3.43143	3.14112	−.15449	−1.092	.2870
ETHNIC	−.30919	.68658	−.05265	−.450	.6571
PSR	.75783	.11850	.77602	6.395	.0000
AGE	−.11163	.17695	−.08690	−.631	.5350
ADTOTAL	−1.58447	2.74104	−.08590	−.578	.5694
(CONSTANT)	99.36390	39.71444		2.502	.0207

Multiple R	.88087
R Square	.77593
Adjusted R Square	.69058
Standard Error	8.26150

Analysis of Variance

	DF	Sum of Squares	Mean Square
Regression	8	4963.50020	620.43753
Residual	21	1433.29980	68.25237

F = 9.09034   Significant F = .0000

sample, is somewhat smaller suggesting a slightly poorer fit of this model for another sample or the population.

DISCUSSION

The results of this study bear out the results of previous research, cited in the introduction, that shows the importance of social support for adequate functioning in the elderly, in this case, in self-reported depression. Preliminary analyses revealed several significant differences between the supported and non-supported groups regarding not only depression scores, but also ADL scores, IADL scores, and PSR scores. In addition, a multiple regression revealed social support to be by far the most powerful predictor of depression in the elderly in this low income housing project. Thus, the area of increasing social supports for elderly residents seems to be well established, certainly for this sample, as the key area for preventive and remedial work for practitioners working with elderly residents in low income housing projects.

In addition since functional disability is frequently encountered in later life it is important to note that the length of stay was longer and the age was higher for supported residents. This might suggest that residents with support can remain independent longer while living in this type of housing–even though their ADL and IADL scores were lower–through the help of family and/or friends.

There were several limitations to this study that might constrain generalizations. First, the size of the sample was relatively small. Second, there were diverse ethnic groups represented in this study and the generalizability of the findings might not be applicable to all groups living on the mainland United States. Third, this study was conducted with low income residents of a housing project for the elderly, so its generalizability to other income groups and to elderly who are not living in housing projects is unknown.

On the other hand, these results do conform to the results of previous research, and may be replicated with other samples in future studies. More research on aging in a variety of living situations is necessary to further understanding of the physical and mental health of the elderly, not only to ease current living conditions and provide more humane and sensitive environments, but to develop programs to prevent premature placement into nursing homes. It is hoped that his study will provide additional impetus for research in this crucial area.

REFERENCES

Arling, G. (1987). Strain, social support, and distress in old age. *Journal of Gerontology, 42*(1), 107-113.

Becker, M.H., & Maiman, L.A. (1980). Strategies for enhancing patient compliance. *Journal of Community Health, 6*, 113-135.

Brock, A.M., & O'Sullivan, P. (1985). A study to determine what variables predict institutionalization of elderly people. *Journal of Advanced Nursing, 10*, 533-537.

Brody, S.J., Poulshock, W., & Masciocchi, C.F. (1978). The family caring unit: A major consideration. *The Gerontologist, 18*, 556-561.

Cassell, J. (1976). The contribution of the social environment to host resistance. *American Journal of Epidemiology, 104*, 107-106.

Chappell, N.L. (1987, June). Household composition and the modified extended family. Paper presented at the annual meeting of the Canadian Sociology and Anthropology Association, Hamilton, Ontario.

Cohen, M.A., Tell, E.J., & Wallack, S. (1986). Client-related risk factors of nursing home entry among elderly adults. *Journal of Gerontology, 41*(1), 785-792.

Corcoran, K., & Fischer, J. (1987). *Measures for clinical practice: A sourcebook.* New York: Macmillan.

David, T.G., Moos, R.H., & Kahn, J.R. (1981). Community integration among elderly residents of sheltered care settings. *American Journal of Community psychology, 9,* 513-526.

Dunlop, B. (1973) *Determinants of long-term care facility utilization by the elderly: An empirical analysis* (Working paper 963-35). Washington, DC: The Urban Institute.

Greenberg, J., & Ginn, A. (1979). A multivariate analysis of the predictors of long-term care placement. *Home Health Care Services Quarterly, 1*(1), 75-99.

Hickey, T. (1975). *Health and aging: The assessment of health and aging.* California: Brooks/Cole.

Hudson, W.W. (1982). *The clinical measurement package: A field manual.* Chicago: Dorsey.

Hughes, S.L., Manheim, L.M., Edelman, P.L., & Conrad, K.J. (1987). Impact of long-term home care on hospital and nursing home use and cost. *Health Services Research, 22*(1), 19-47.

Kahn, R.L., Wetherington, E., & Ingersoll-Dayton, B. (1990). Social support and social support networks: Determinants, effects, and interactions. In R. Abeles (Ed.), *Implications of the life-span perspective for social psychology* (pp. 139-165). New York: Erlbaum.

Kane, R.A., & Kane R.L. (1984). Assessing the elderly: A practical guide to measurement. Massachusetts: Lexington.

Katz, S., Ford, A.B., Moskowitz, R.W., Jackson, B.A., & Jaffee, M.W. (1963). Studies of illness in the aged. The index of ADL: A standardized measure of biological and psychosocial function. *Journal of the American Medical Association, 185.*

Katz, S., Hedrick, S., & Henderson, N. (1979). The measurement of long-term care needs and impact. *Health and Medical Care Services Review, 2,* 2-21.

Krause, N. (1990). Perceived health problems, formal and informal support, and life satisfaction among older adults. *Journal of Gerontology, 45*(5), 193-205.

Lemke, S., & Moos, R.H. (1986). Quality of residential settings for elderly adults. *Journal of Gerontology, 41*(2), 268-276.

Lowenthal, M.F., & Haven, C. (1968). Interaction and adaptation: Intimacy as a critical variable. *American Sociology Review, 35,* 20-31.

Macken, C. (1986). A profile of functionally impaired elderly persons living in the community. *Health Care Financing Review, 7*(4), 33-49.

Maguire, L. (1980). The interface of social workers with personal networks. *Social Work with Groups, 3,* 39-49.

McAuley, W., & Prohaska, T. (1982). Professional recommendations for long-term care placement: A comparison of two groups of institutionally vulnerable elderly. *Home Health Care Services Quarterly, 2*(3), 51-57.

McCoy, J., & Edwards, B. (1981). Contextual and sociodemographic antecedents of institutionalization among aged welfare recipients. *Medical Care, 19,* 907-921.

Morris, J.N., Sherwood, S., & Gutkin, C.E. (1988). Inst-Risk II: An approach to forecasting relative risk of future institutional placement. *Health Services Research, 23*(4), 511-536.

Palmore, E. (1976). Total chance of institutionalization among the aged. *The Gerontologist, 16,* 504-507.

Peters, G.R., & Kaiser, M.A. (1985). The role of friends and neighbors in providing social support. In W.J. Sauer & R.T. Coward (Eds.), *Social support networks and the care of the elderly* (pp. 123-158). New York: Springer.

Shapiro, E., & Tate, R. (1988). Who is really at risk of institutionalization? *The Gerontologist, 28,* 237-245.

Smallegan, M. (1985). There was nothing else to do: Needs for care before nursing home admission. *The Gerontologist, 25,* 364-369.

Smyer, M. (1980). The differential usage of services by impaired elderly. *Journal of Gerontology, 35*(2), 249-255.

Turner, R.J., Frankel, B.G., & Levin, D.M. (1983). Social support: Conceptualization, measurement, and implications for mental health. *Research in community and mental health 3,* 67-111.

Ulbrich, P.M., & Warheit, G.J. (1989). Social support, stress, and psychological distress among older black and white adults. *Journal of Aging and Health,* 1(3), 286-305.

Vicente, L., Wiley, J.A., & Carrington, R.A. (1979). The risk of institutionalization before death. *The Gerontologist,* 19, 361-367.

Wan, T.H., & Weissert, W.G. (1981). Social support networks, patient status and institutionalization. *Research on Aging, 3*(2), 240-256.

Weissert, W., & Cready, C. (1989). Toward a model for improved targeting of aged at risk of institutionalization. *Health Services Research 24*(4), 487-510.

Attitudes of Housing Professionals Toward Residential Options for the Elderly

Carla C. Earhart

SUMMARY. In response to the need to house the older population, a variety of alternatives have surfaced. However, these have been met with disparate responses–favorable from older consumers, but negative from some housing professionals. This research was conducted to better understand the attitudes of housing professionals toward various alternatives for the elderly. Randomly selected housing professionals practicing in a Midwestern county responsed to a mailed questionnaire addressing their knowledge of the older population and attitudes toward senior housing options. Results show few respondents had accurate information about seniors. Additionally, while housing professionals were highly aware of traditional housing alternatives, they were less familiar with more innovative options. Further findings reflect that some groups of housing professionals are significantly less likely than others to support innovative housing options. Suggestions are made for developing educational programs for housing professionals. *[Article copies available for a fee from The Haworth Document Delivery Service: 1-800-342-9678. E-mail address: getinfo@ haworthpressinc.com]*

KEYWORDS. Housing alternatives, discrepancies between customers and housing professionals, professionals lack knowledge of alternatives, failure of professionals to support innovative options, need for educational programs for professionals

---

Carla C. Earhart, PhD, CFCS, is Associate Professor, Department of Family & Consumer Sciences, Ball State University, Muncie, IN 47306.

Funding for this project was provided by a grant from the Office of Academic Research & Sponsored Programs, Ball State University.

[Haworth co-indexing entry note]: "Attitudes of Housing Professionals Toward Residential Options for the Elderly." Earhart, Carla C. Co-published simultaneously in *Journal of Housing for the Elderly* (The Haworth Press, Inc.) Vol. 13, No. 1/2, 1999, pp. 65-78; and: *Making Aging in Place Work* (ed: Leon A. Pastalan) The Haworth Press, Inc., 1999, pp. 65-78. Single or multiple copies of this article are available for a fee from The Haworth Document Delivery Service [1-800-342-9678, 9:00 a.m. - 5:00 p.m. (EST). E-mail address: getinfo@haworthpressinc.com].

INTRODUCTION

Housing alternatives that meet the diverse needs of the increasingly older population have been conceived, but resistance has been met by housing professionals. While research related to innovative housing for the elderly has been conducted from the perspective of the elderly resident, little is known about the attitudes of housing professionals toward such alternatives, except that they are negative. Additional research is needed to more fully understand the perspective of housing professionals who are in a position to provide appropriate housing for older persons. Results can be used to educate housing professionals on the housing needs of the elderly, thus improving the availability of appropriate housing options.

REVIEW OF LITERATURE

The elderly population is not homogeneous (AARP, 1989; Soldo, 1982). Their life histories, experiences, attitudes, and preferences coupled with a wide range of demographic characteristics emphasize the fact that no single policy, program, or provision can meet their individual needs. This is certainly true with regards to housing.

The acknowledgment of this diversity of those age 65 and older is opening up more housing alternatives for older people (Atchley, 1988). Yet, housing appropriate to individual needs remains in short supply with at least 20 percent of elderly persons in inappropriate housing (Guidon, 1983/84).

According to Lawton (1985), the majority of older persons live in their own single-family detached unit in a community setting. This is the preferred option and the most independent type of living arrangement, but may not meet the needs of all elderly people. Many others live in mobile homes, senior apartments, or retirement condominiums. Only about five percent live in dependent care. It is likely that many of these do not need the full services of a nursing home, but without other alternatives, are forced to resort to such arrangements.

In response to this growing need, a variety of housing alternatives have surfaced. These include the accessory apartment, granny flat, shared housing, group housing, life care community, and reverse annuity mortgage, as well as many others. Each is designed for a specific group of the varied elderly population.

The growth in housing alternatives for the elderly has been met with disparate responses. On the one hand, older persons themselves report a high level of interest in such specialized arrangements (Hare & Haske, 1983/84; Pollack & Malakoff, 1984). On the other hand, housing providers contend that such alternatives have negative aspects that make them impractical for additional consideration (Ehrlich, 1986; Hare, 1985; Hopperton, 1986).

Patrick Hare (1984), a pioneer in innovative living arrangements for the elderly, maintains that housing providers are leery about these housing alternatives because they are unfamiliar with such innovations. He suggests that lack of awareness and knowledge about such housing creates ignorance about their true value. Additionally, such negative attitudes may be related to stereotypical information about elderly persons. However, research to support these claims is not available.

As the number of and variation in elderly people continue to increase, so too has the need for improving their primary lifespace—the home. Efforts to increase the diversity and quality of housing opportunities have been met with opposition from housing professionals who control the housing supply. Such opposition may be related to lack of awareness and/or lack of knowledge related to the elderly and their housing situation. Research is needed to more fully understand the attitudes of housing professionals toward housing alternatives for the elderly.

PURPOSE AND OBJECTIVES

The purpose of this research is to more fully understand the attitudes of housing professionals toward various housing alternatives. Specific variables to be studied include:

1. knowledge about the older population;
2. awareness of housing alternatives;
3. support for housing alternatives; and
4. differences in support for alternatives according to professional group.

METHODOLOGY

The population used in this study includes housing professionals practicing in a Midwestern county, comprised of home builders, interior designers, city planners, developers, real estate agents and appraisers, architects, and mortgage lenders. A random sample of each group was chosen from business listings in the area telephone directory resulting in 57 potential respondents. Incorporated into the research instrument was a true/false quiz of general information related to the older population, adapted from AARP (1989). The quiz was followed by a series of Likert scales querying respondents' awareness of and support for 23 senior housing options. Space was provided to write in comments pertaining to perceived benefits and detriments of each respondent, including age, gender, years in the housing profession, area of professional practice, and frequency of contact with other persons. A set of definitions accompanied each survey to assist respondents in understanding unfamiliar terms.[1]

Data was collected by mail using Dillman's (1978) Total Design Method. This procedure included sending the mail questionnaire with a self-addressed stamped reply envelope, which was followed up by a reminder postcard. The resulting response rate was 37 percent.

RESULTS

Characteristics of Respondents

As shown in Table 1, information from the participants reveal that respondent age ranged from 33 to 75 years, with a mean of about 51 years. Replies were fairly well divided between male and female respondents. Respondents represented the full range of professional practice groups within the housing profession–architects, mortgage lenders, real estate agents and appraisers. Years in the housing profession ranged from less than one to over 20; over half had been in the business for 16 years or more.

When asked about the level of contact with persons age 65 and over, the majority of respondents indicated frequent associations.

---

1. A list of definitions used in the study may be obtained from the author.

TABLE 1. Characteristics of Respondents

	frequency	percent
Age:		
less than 35	1	5.6
35-44	4	22.3
45-54	5	27.9
55-64	6	33.4
65 and over	2	11.2
Gender:		
male	11	55.0
female	9	45.0
Area of Specialization:		
Architect	2	10.0
Builder	2	10.0
City Planner	4	20.0
Developer	2	10.0
Interior Designer	2	10.0
Mortgage Lender	2	10.0
Real Estate Agent	4	20.0
Real Estate Appraiser	2	10.0
Years in Practice:		
less than 1 year	1	5.0
1-5 years	1	5.0
6-10 years	2	10.0
11-15 years	7	35.0
16-20 years	1	5.0
more than 20 years	8	40.0
Contact with Elderly:		
none	0	0.0
very little	0	0.0
some	5	25.0
frequently	8	40.0
on a daily basis	7	35.0

However, such contact did not necessarily equate with accurate knowledge about older persons.

Knowledge of the Older Population

Ten true and false statements adapted from a 1989 AARP publication comprised the knowledge quiz on the elderly population. Statements included facts that directly or indirectly impact the older persons' residential environment. Table 2 provides details about the statements and the accuracy of the housing professionals' responses.

On the quiz, nearly all of the respondents has correct information about the size of the elderly population and the amount of money older persons spend on health care. About two-thirds of the sample responded accurately to statements regarding older persons' marital status, residential mobility, educational attainment, tenure status, housing quality, and personal assistance needs. Statements pertaining to the net worth of elderly households and the percentage of older persons in nursing homes were answered incorrectly by over half of the housing professionals.

When quiz responses were totaled for each participant, the results indicated that less than five percent achieved perfect scores. Less than half of the respondents scored at 70 percent of above. Table 3 provides additional details about the quiz scores.

Familiarity with Housing Options

Participants were asked to indicate their level of familiarity with 23 senior housing options on a Likert scale ranging from 1 (never heard of it) to 8 (am currently living in one). Housing options were grouped into four categories: structure types, living arrangements, methods of acquisition, and specialized assistance programs. Findings are presented in Table 4.

Mean scores on the familiarity scale indicated housing professionals were quite familiar with traditional structure types such as Single-Family Detached Houses and Apartments. Respondents were less familiar with Mobile Homes, Duplexes, and Townhouses.

Respondents' familiarity with various living arrangements ranged from a high of x = 7.10 for Independent Living to a low of x = 2.19 for Granny Flats. Other mean scores for living arrangements indicate,

TABLE 2. Knowledge of the Older Population

Statement	Correct Responses	
	frequency	percent
The older population represents less than 10 percent of the U.S. population. (False)	20	95.2
Older men are more likely to be married than older women. (True)	16	76.2
Approximately 15 percent of those age 65 and older are living in nursing homes. (False)	10	47.6
Older persons are less likely to move than any other age group. (True)	15	71.4
The median net worth of older households is significantly higher than the national average. (True)	8	38.1
About half of those people age 65 and older have completed high school. (True)	14	66.7
Elderly households are more likely to be renters than home owners. (False)	14	66.7
Housing of older persons is generally older and less adequate than housing of other age groups. (True)	15	71.4
Older persons spend about the same amount of money on health care as younger persons. (False)	19	90.5
About one-quarter of older persons need assistance with personal care and/or home management activities. (True)	15	71.4

TABLE 3. Total Quiz Scores

Number of Correct Responses (maximum score of 10)	frequency	percent
0	1	4.8
1	0	0.0
2	0	0.0
3	1	4.8
4	0	0.0
5	0	0.0
6	3	14.3
7	7	33.3
8	6	28.6
9	2	9.5
10	1	4.8

again, that housing professionals were much more familiar with traditional living arrangements.

Mean familiarity scores for methods of acquisition revealed participants were well acquainted with traditional Fee Simple Ownership, but much less familiar with non-traditional Cooperative Ownership. Housing professionals were somewhat aware of Condominium Ownership and Renting.

When asked about familiarity with specialized assistance programs, housing professionals were not well acquainted with any of the benefit plans. Mean familiarity scores ranged from a high of $x = 4.10$ for Subsidized Housing to a low of $x = 3.10$ for Property Tax Assistance.

Support for Housing Options

Housing professionals were asked to disclose their support for the 23 senior housing options on a Likert scale ranging from 1 (definitely would not support) to 5 (definitely would support). Findings are illustrated in Table 5.

Respondents were very supportive of two structure types for older persons–Single-Family Detached Houses and Duplexes. Although not as strongly, they were overall supportive of Mobile, Townhouses, and Apartments.

TABLE 4. Familiarity with Housing Options

	Mean Score 1 = low; 8 = high
Structure Types:	
Single-family detached house	7.60
Mobile home	5.20
Duplex	5.41
Townhouse	4.95
Apartment	6.15
Living Arrangements:	
Independent living	7.10
Living with children	4.95
Shared housing	3.44
Accessory apartment	3.81
Group housing	3.48
Granny flat	2.19
Nursing home	4.67
Life care community	3.10
Methods of Acquisition:	
Fee simple ownership	7.10
Condominium ownership	5.25
Cooperative ownership	2.79
Renting	5.76
Housing Assistance Programs:	
Home-provided services	3.86
Subsidized housing	4.10
Home weatherization/repair	3.71
Property tax assistance	3.10
Capital gains exclusion	3.81
Reverse annuity mortgage	3.52

Mean support scores for living arrangements indicated housing professionals were more supportive of Life Care Communities and Independent Living. Other living arrangements the respondents would support but to a lesser extent include Shared Housing, Accessory Apartments, Group Housing, Granny Flats, and Nursing Homes. Housing professionals were not supportive of the options of elderly persons Living with Children.

TABLE 5. Support for Housing Options

	Mean Score 1 = low; 5 = high
Structure Types:	
Single-family detached house	4.20
Mobile home	3.26
Duplex	4.11
Townhouse	3.24
Apartment	3.86
Living Arrangements:	
Independent living	4.10
Living with children	3.00
Shared housing	3.29
Accessory apartment	3.76
Group housing	3.29
Granny flat	3.22
Nursing home	3.62
Life care community	4.35
Methods of Acquisition:	
Fee simple ownership	4.40
Condominium ownership	4.52
Cooperative ownership	3.00
Renting	3.86
Housing Assistance Programs:	
Home-provided services	4.14
Subsidized housing	3.48
Home weatherization/repair	3.86
Property tax assistance	3.20
Capital gains exclusion	4.60
Reverse annuity mortgage	3.75

Mean support scores for the methods in which older persons acquire housing indicate housing professionals lend more support to Condominium Ownership. Renting is somewhat supported by the respondents. Overall, Cooperative Ownership is not supported by the housing professionals in the study.

When queried about specialized programs to assist elderly persons with their housing needs, respondents were overall supportive of the options. Capital Gains Exclusion and Home-Provided Services received the greatest support. Housing professionals were also supportive of Subsidized Housing, Home Weatherization/Repair, Property Tax Assistance, and Reserve Annuity Mortgages.

Differences in Support by Professional Group

The appearance of housing professionals' support for the various housing options may be deceiving until analyzed for differences by professional group. Using One-Way Analysis of Variance, statistically significant differences (at $p = .05$) were found in support for Apartments, Life-Care Communities, Renting, Cooperative Ownership, Home-Provided Services and Home Weatherization/Repair. Findings are illustrated in Table 6.

Using the Scheffe Procedure, differences in support for the senior housing options were delineated by professional group. Apartments were, not surprisingly, supported by city planners, but also by real estate agents, appraisers, and mortgage lenders. Support for this option was not given by architects, interior designers, developers, or builders. Life Care Communities were supported by all except real estate agents and appraisers.

Only city planners gave any support to Cooperative Ownership. Renting was supported by all except real estate agents and appraisers. Home-Provided Services and Home Weatherization/Repair were supported by all housing professional excluding builders.

SUMMARY

Although housing options that meet the diverse needs of the aging population have been conceived, additional information was needed to understand the value of these options from the perspective of housing professionals who are in a position to make such options available or create barriers to the supply. To fill this gap, this research has sought to determine housing professionals' knowledge about older persons, awareness of and support for myriad options, and whether there are differences in support among the various specializations within the housing industry.

Results of the aging quiz indicate that while few achieved perfect scores, many housing professionals, nonetheless, are reasonably knowl-

TABLE 6. Analysis of Variance: Differences in Support by Professional Group

	F ratio	p value
Structure Types:		
Single-family detached	2.0579	.1411
Mobile Home	1.4654	.2697
Duplex	0.1993	.9348
Townhouse	1.9741	.1503
Apartment	4.6714	.0120*
Living Arrangements:		
Independent living	0.1071	.9782
Living with children	0.1043	.9793
Shared housing	1.7500	.2101
Accessory apartment	0.9581	.4585
Group housing	1.1932	.3540
Granny flat	1.4375	.2811
Nursing home	0.2422	.9099
Life care community	3.6003	.0413*
Methods of Acquisition:		
Fee simple ownership	0.3142	.8637
Condominium ownership	0.9524	.4520
Cooperative ownership	0.3142	.8637
Renting	3.5779	.0457*
Housing Assistance Programs:		
Home-provided services	7.1667	.0020*
Subsidized housing	1.2994	.3146
Home weatherization/repair	4.3125	.0161*
Property tax assistance	2.5840	.0828
Capital gains exclusion	1.5809	.2339
Reverse annuity mortgage	3.0428	.0533

*statistically significant at $p = .05$

edgeable about older persons' needs and characteristics. However, caution must be used in interpreting this information. While these overall high scores are welcome news, more substantial information comes from analyzing the specific questions that were most often missed on the quiz. Respondents failed to realize that older persons do, in fact, have considerable asset accumulation. Such assets could be sold and used for housing-related purchases. Many housing professionals were also in error in the percentage of older persons residing in nursing homes, perceiving it to be much higher than the actual percentage. This may indicate that housing professionals are unaware of the number of older persons who are in need of community-based housing, which could be a niche market for professionals in the housing industry.

Of the 23 senior housing options presented, housing professionals were familiar with only about half of them. They were much more aware of traditional housing options for the elderly (single-family detached houses, nursing homes, and fee simple ownership). Professionals in the field report little awareness of more innovative options—granny flats, life care communities, cooperative ownership, and reverse annuity mortgages. Such options are the ones reported to have the highest level of interest by the elderly themselves (Pollack & Malakoff, 1984).

Excluding cooperative ownership and living with children, housing professionals overall were surprisingly supportive of the remaining 21 senior housing options presented. This was true even for the housing options that were relatively unfamiliar to the respondents. Perhaps they do, in fact, support myriad housing alternatives for the elderly, once they are familiarized with the alternatives available.

As previously noted, there were differences in support of some of the senior housing options among the various specializations in the housing field. City planners appear to be overall more supportive of diversity in housing than the other professional groups. Real estate agents and builders were less supportive of diverse housing options. Written comments indicate that these two groups tend to support those senior housing options perceived to enhance their business. Unless the housing option required new construction, which would benefit the builder, or relocating, which would benefit the real estate agent, these housing professionals were less likely to support it.

CONCLUSIONS

The results of this investigation suggest that housing professionals lack important information about older persons that may influence the ability of the housing industry to provide appropriate housing options. Further, professionals in the field are unaware of the growing number of innovative housing alternatives designed to meet the unique needs of the older population. After becoming more familiar with the alternatives, housing professionals are more supportive of the various housing options. Support increases when housing professionals perceive their own business will be enhanced by such options.

To improve their knowledge about the older population and increase their awareness of the myriad housing options available, educational programs need to be implemented. Such programs will need to stress not only the benefit of the housing options to the elderly residents, but to the housing professionals as well. To improve participation, programs could be sponsored or endorsed by the professional associations in the housing field with continuing education credits available.

Although the findings of this exploratory study shed light on an area lacking research-based information, the results cannot be considered conclusive or exhaustive. This study involved only 21 respondents in a small geographic location. More comprehensive studies are needed to improve the size and geographic diversity of the sample.

REFERENCES

American Association of Retired Persons. (1993). *A Profile of Older Americans.* Washington, DC: AARP.

Dillman, D.A. (1978). *Mail and Telephone Surveys: The Total Design Method.* New York: Wiley-Interscience.

Atchley, R.C. (1988). *Social Forces and Aging.* Belmont, CA: Wadsworth Publishing Co.

Ehrlich, P. (1986). Hotels, rooming houses, shared housing, and other housing options for the marginal elderly. In R.J. Newcomer, M.P. Lawton, and T.O. Byerts, (Eds.), *Housing an Aging Society.* New York: Van Nostrand Reinhold.

Guidon, E. (1983/84). A new feature on the housing horizon. *Aging, 342,* 9-11.

Hare, P. (1984). ECHO housing. In L. Hubbard, (Ed.), *Housing Options for Older Americans.* Washington Association of Retired Persons.

Hare, P. (1985). Accessory apartments: Who can afford to market the concept? *Generations, 3,* 44-45.

Hare, P. and Haske, M. (1983/84). Innovative living arrangements, *Aging, 342,* 3-8.

Hopperton, R. (1986). Land-use regulations for the elderly. In R.J. Newcomer, M.P. Lawton, and T.O. Byerts, (Eds.), *Housing an Aging Society.* New York: Van Nostrand Reinhold.

Lawton, M.P. (1985). Housing and living environment of older people. In R.H. Binstock and E. Shanas, (Eds.), *Handbook of Aging and the Social Sciences.* New York: Van Nostrand Reinhold.

Pollack, P.B. and Malakoff, L.Z. (1984). Housing for the elderly: Five new ideas. *Consumer Close-Ups.* Ithaca, NY: Cornell University, Department of Consumer Economics and Housing.

Mental Health Needs and Supportive Services for Elderly and Disabled Residents

Jungwee Park

Jean Burritt Robertson

SUMMARY. This study longitudinally assesses the impact that the provision of supportive services has on the mental well-being of the elderly and disabled population living in independent housing developments. The results indicate that the use of supportive services by the mentally ill allowed them to overcome initial lower functional status and achieve a level of mental functioning virtually similar to that of the total resident population. Thus, it is argued that independent living facilities with supportive services can certainly be a successful and cost effective model for a number of frail elderly and mentally ill residents. *[Article copies available for a fee from The Haworth Document Delivery Service: 1-800-342-9678. E-mail address: getinfo@haworthpressinc.com]*

KEYWORDS. Longitudinal assessment, support services, well-being, elderly and disabled residents, mentally ill residents, cost effective model

INTRODUCTION

The proportion of elderly in America will continue to increase substantially over the next few decades. It will account for more than

Jungwee Park, PhD, is affiliated with the Department of Sociology, Humboldt State University, Arcata, CA 95521. Jean Burritt Robertson, MA, is Research Coordinator, Rhode Island Housing & Mortgage Finance Corporation, 44 Washington Street, Providence, RI 02903.

The authors would like to thank Dr. Phil Brown for his helpful comments and criticisms.

[Haworth co-indexing entry note]: "Mental Health Needs and Supportive Services for Elderly and Disabled Residents." Park, Jungwee, and Jean Burritt Robertson. Co-published simultaneously in *Journal of Housing for the Elderly* (The Haworth Press, Inc.) Vol. 13, No. 1/2, 1999, pp. 79-91; and: *Making Aging in Place Work* (ed: Leon A. Pastalan) The Haworth Press, Inc., 1999, pp. 79-91. Single or multiple copies of this article are available for a fee from The Haworth Document Delivery Service [1-800-342-9678, 9:00 a.m. - 5:00 p.m. (EST). E-mail address: getinfo@haworthpressinc.com].

20 percent of the population by 2030; the number of the "frail" elderly, those 75 years old and older, will also be as great as 9.2 percent (U.S. Bureau of the Census, 1993). As of 1992, in Rhode Island, 15.2 percent of the state population is already 65 years or older. It is also estimated that by 2020, 22 percent of Rhode Islanders will be senior citizens and the number of the frail elderly will virtually quadruple compared to the figure of 1960 (RI Division of Planning, 1992; 1993). Such rapid aging of American society deserves sociological attention since the changing age structure affects every aspect of the social and economic life of people of all ages. Population aging is not simply of societal interest to the old. To be specific, the aging of the population has raised questions about increased demands on the health care, housing, income security, transportation and social service systems (Marshall et al., 1987). Thus, issues related to the elderly and aging, are increasingly drawing national attention.

Housing for the frail elderly is a major social concern. Many of the older retirees can no longer manage in their own homes due to their functional limitations. The process of aging results in physical and cognitive frailties which tend to get worse over time. Many elderly need some assistance with the activities of daily life but are still far too independent to require placement in a nursing home or similar institutional facility (Monk and Kaye, 1991). In addition, given the high cost of institutionalization, and the issues of self-determination, there is growing demand for cost effective housing alternatives which allow greater independence. According to Carlin and Mansberg (1984), over three million elderly in the United States are in need of some form of assisted living. Without a range of alternatives, a number of elderly end up in nursing homes prematurely. Heumann and Boldy (1982) claim that between 20 and 30 percent of those now in nursing homes could live independently if proper assistance were available.

Coincident with the emergence of focus on housing arrangements for the elderly, the housing patterns and treatment of mentally ill and disabled persons were also undergoing rapid changes with the deinstitutionalization policy. Certainly, it can be argued that cost is a paramount interest in most of the decisions surrounding change. A variety of non-institutional housing models have been introduced as alternatives to nursing home and hospital placement (Silverman, 1987). One of the models is private housing with supportive services available as needed. According to a study conducted by the government, support services for frail elderly or handicapped persons in government assisted housing not only delay the need for a move to nursing homes but the cost of a support services program was found to be about one-third the cost of institutionalized care (National Association of Housing and Redevelopment Officials, 1985).

While these studies, especially government reports have found that supportive services which allow the elderly and disabled to remain in an independent living situation are cost effective, almost none of them have carefully analyzed the impact of supportive services on the health or quality of life of the elderly and disabled residents. The present study focuses on the issue missing from most previous studies: the impact of services on the mental health and quality of life for both elderly and mentally ill residents. Mental functioning is one of the most significant indicators of the quality of life. Unfortunately, it is known that a very high proportion of elderly people suffer from various mental health problems in this country.

The elderly are generally considered more likely than younger age groups to suffer from psychiatric impairment (D'Arcy, 1987). A variety of previous epidemiological studies have shown higher prevalence rates of psychiatric disorder among the elderly (George et al., 1988; Neugebauer, 1980; Neugebauer, Dohrenwend, and Dohrenwend, 1980; Blazer, 1980). The average incidence of psychosis increases with age, with the increase in new cases most marked after age 70 (World Health Organization, 1959; Butler, 1975; Jaco, 1960; Kay and Bergmann, 1980; Cohen, 1977, 1980). Moreover, mental health problems among the elderly, like depression, are prone to be undiagnosed or misdiagnosed. Because depression may be connected to age-specific stressful life events such as loss of spouse, declining health, loss of income and independence, and diminished social supports, depression among the aged may present itself in forms unlike those found in younger age groups (Cheah, 1978).

Higher suicide rates among the aged are also indicative of the increased incidence of psychological despair among the elderly (D'Arcy, 1987). In fact, unrecognized psychiatric illness, depression, especially–not living conditions–is the major factor in old-age suicide (cf., O'Neal, 1966). National statistics show that older people, who made up 12.7 percent of the U.S. population in 1992, commit 21 percent of the officially recognized suicides. Their rate, 20.1 suicides per 100,000 people, is about 60 percent higher than that of the nation as a whole (U.S. Bureau of the Census, 1993). Furthermore, such a high suicide rate is only a part of the truth. Suicide attributed to the elderly tends to be drastically under-reported. Many suicidal old people take a slow, indirect way out by starving themselves or not taking necessary medication (Osgood, Brant and Lipman, 1991). In a sense, the success rate of suicide increases with age (Lester, 1994; D'Arcy, 1987).

Rhode Island Housing and Mortgage Finance Corporation, the chief sponsor of this research, has been a pioneer in providing supportive services since 1986 to elderly and disabled residents in the 108 housing developments it finances and monitors. It was one of the first state housing agencies in the country to aid in the deinstitutionalization of the state's mentally ill, and developmentally disabled residents by providing independent housing in its developments as early as 1980. In 1988, the Corporation received a grant from the Robert Wood Johnson Foundation to develop a more comprehensive, well-organized, and flexible approach to the delivery of supportive services for elderly and disabled residents. Twelve developments were chosen for this pilot program.

The research began with a survey of residents in twelve housing developments for the elderly and disabled. A total of 1,294 units were occupied in the twelve developments and 600 residents were selected for the sample. According to this survey, as many as 34 percent of the residents were reporting problems with sleep; 29 percent felt depressed; and 28 percent reported feelings of anxiety and nervousness. The majority of respondents were not getting any help for these problems, and interest was high for a service to deal with mental health problems. Thirty-seven reported a willingness to use a free medically supervised service that helped people with problems with sleep, memory, mood, or anxiety.

The goal of this paper is to assess the impact of the provision of supportive services on the mental health of the residents in elderly housing developments. In order to assess the impact of services, we conducted a longitudinal analysis, in which all residents receiving services were interviewed twice, at six month intervals. A total of 205 residents were studied before and again six months after receiving support services. The study focused primarily on determining the extent to which receipt of services resulted in meaningful changes in both the metal health and the quality of life for residents.

METHODS

Evaluation of alternative housing and health care programs has become an area of specialization in its own right. Strategies for altering the health status of the elderly and disabled require a technology for first assessing the health status and then detecting increments of progress. The mental, physical and social well-being of individuals are very closely interrelated, making it necessary to use multi-dimensional health assessments. According to Kane and Kane (1981), measures of functional status that examine the ability to function independently despite disease, physical and mental disability, and social deprivation are the most useful overall indicators.

Assessment Tools

To obtain multi-dimensional health assessments as Kane and Kane suggested, we reviewed classes of measurement such as measures of functional status (Katz, Hedrick, and Henderson, 1979; Goga and Hambacher, 1977); subjective well-being or happiness (Larson, 1978; George, 1979); life adjustment (Graney and Graney, 1973); mental functioning or depression (Gallagher, Thompson, and Levy, 1980; Salzman et al., 1972a, b; Raskin and Jarvik, 1979); and quality of life (George and Bearon, 1980). Based on such review of the literature, consultation with experts in the field, and the need for an easily administered and relatively short assessment, several existing and well tested assessment tools were combined into an overall assessment. The tool was intended to examine several aspects of health and well-being. The basic tool used has several components to measure areas of mental health and well-being. It includes cognitive functioning, affective functioning, and psycho-social well-being.

Area of Assessment	Measurement Tool
Psycho-Social Well-Being	UCLA Designed Survey
Cognitive Functioning	Mini Mental Health Status Exam
Affective Functioning	UCLA–Functional Status Questionnaire

Data

This study is based primarily upon 410 cases of interview derived data. Residents of the twelve elderly housing developments in Rhode

Island were interviewed. These cases include 205 initial and 205 follow-up interviews. Follow-up interviews were conducted six months after the provision of services. To see if there would be a measurable effect resulting from the service provision on mental health, the research makes use of two sets of results: one from the initial interview group, the other from the follow-up group. By using this longitudinal approach, it is hypothesized that measurable changes would occur after the provision of services.

The data-set also includes a total of 44 mentally ill residents (before and after the provision of services altogether). These residents either reported themselves as mentally ill or were known by interviewers to be mentally disabled. In most cases, self-reporting and interviewer knowledge were consistent. The research compares this mentally ill group with the entire resident group to see if the impact of the services on mental health varies for the two groups.

Variables

The presence or absence of support services is the independent variable. Supportive services offered in the housing developments include heavy and light household chores, personal care services, food preparation, and shopping. The major service used was household chore service which accounted for about 64 percent of the services performed. This usually consisted of cleaning showers, tubs, refrigerators, and floors and changing bed linens. Laundry was the next highest use area accounting for 24 percent of the services used. Shopping accounted for 8 percent of services, followed by personal care at 3 percent and food preparation at 2 percent. The major personal care use was for help with hair shampooing. In addition, homemakers often helped residents with medications primarily by setting up their medications for the week in a way that prompted residents to take them and allowed for easy determination of consumption which was very helpful for those with poor recall.

The level of mental functioning served as the dependent variable. The dependent variable was measured by three indicators including cognitive (COG), affective (AFF), and psycho-social well-being (PSW) scores. The standard mini-mental status examination underlies cognitive scores; affective scores concern residents' psychological state, for example, how depressed (or cheerful) they are; psycho-social well-being is a measurement consisting of questions on sociability with others. Compared are mental health functioning between the mentally ill and all residents before and after the provision of the services.

RESULTS

Table 1 shows the overall mean scores of the three dependent variables. Not surprisingly, mentally ill residents were evaluated as having lower cognitive and affective scores. Mean differences between total sample and the mentally ill were statistically significant (at 99 and 95% level, respectively). However, the two population groups did not have any discrepancy in scores of psycho-social well-being. The greatest differences in the two population groups occurred in the indicators more strictly tied to mental status.

Tables 2 and 3 indicate mean scores on cognitive, affective and psycho-social well-being evaluations before and after the provision of supportive services. As expected, mean differences before the services

TABLE 1. Overall Mean Scores

	COG	AFF	PSW
Mentally Ill	12.9	18.7	23.6
Total	16.1	20.2	23.6
Mean Difference	3.2***	1.5**	0.0

**Significant at 95% level
***Significant at 99% level

TABLE 2. Mean Scores Before the Provision of Services

	COG	AFF	PSW
Mentally Ill	11.6	18.0	23.3
Total	16.7	19.8	23.9
Mean Difference	5.1***	1.8**	0.6

**Significant at 95% level
***Significant at 99% level

TABLE 3. Mean Scores After the Provision of Services

	COG	AFF	PSW
Mentally Ill	14.1	19.5	23.9
Total	15.3	20.7	23.1
Mean Difference	1.2	1.2	− .6

were offered are statistically meaningful, except for scores of psychosocial well-being. Clearly, Table 2 follows the pattern of Table 1 for the entire population with greater mean differences.

Table 3, however, indicates a different pattern from the previous tables. Mean differences between the mentally ill and overall population are reduced so strikingly that none of the differences are significant. The psychosocial well-being score of the mentally ill is even higher than that of the total population after the provision of services. These results mean that the supportive services are especially helpful to mentally ill residents while also improving aspects of mental health for the elderly in general. The results indicate that the use of supportive services by the mentally ill allowed them to overcome initially lower functional scores and achieve a level of mental functioning virtually similar to that of the total resident population.

Figures 1, 2, and 3 graphically present the positive impact resulting from the provision of supportive services on the status of the mentally ill. For cognitive scores, the initial difference reduced almost to zero after the services were given (Figure 1); for affective scores, the difference reduced greatly although some discrepancy still exists; for psychosocial well-being scores, a "cross-over" was witnessed.

As the results indicate, the mentally ill residents had far more remarkable increases in cognitive, affective and psychosocial well-being scores. This implies that the provision of services is even more important for the mentally ill who started off with relatively low scores. Improvements in mental health may be directly related to support providers' reminders to clients to take their prescribed medications. Help with medications is a common service provided.

The overall improvement in outlook is extremely remarkable. The provision of services may alleviate a great deal of worry about getting things done, for the mentally ill, as it did for the elderly. The mentally

FIGURE 1. Cognitive Scores Before and After Services for Mentally Ill and All Residents

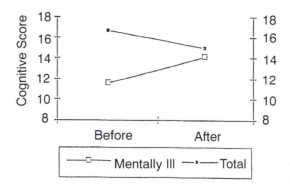

FIGURE 2. Affective Scores Before and After Services for Mentally Ill and All Residents

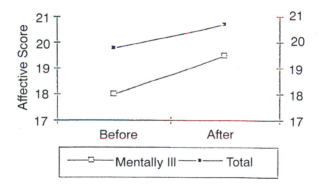

ill, who are a minority in the housing developments, and many of whom were fairly recently deinstitutionalized, may also be suffering from the lack of human interaction. Interaction with the provider could be an important, if unintended, beneficial side effect of service provision.

DISCUSSION

The findings point out two meaningful effects from the provision of supportive services on the well-being of mentally ill and frail elderly

FIGURE 3. Psychosocial Well-Being Before and After Services for Mentally III and All Residents

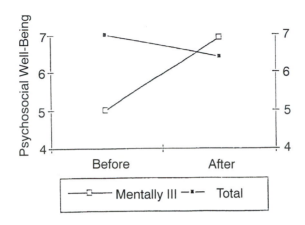

residents living independently: first, in the long run, the services help people by freeing them from the fear of being institutionalized. Indeed, subsequent face-to-face interviews with residents indicated that before services they were more worried about how things would get done. More importantly, a majority mentioned that if the services were not available, no one else would help them and, as a result, they feared institutionalization and nursing home placement. Second, in the short run, the mentally ill and frail elderly residents receiving services showed marked improvements in their quality of life due to better nutrition, as a result of help with meal preparation; and closer monitoring of prescription medicines. Those are assured by the supportive service providers.

Overall, it is believed that support services, especially for the mentally ill should be a mandatory component of all plans for deinstitutionlization because the services impressively improve the mental and social functioning of this population with relatively low costs. The services also appear to reduce significantly the chance for serious regression of mental health and subsequent need for reinstitutionalization.

Among the elderly with high health care expenses (over $2,000 annually), nursing home costs were responsible for over 80 percent of their expenditures. Fully half of all nursing home expenses are paid by residents' and their families' personal savings. Just over 47 percent of these costs are paid by the Federal Government, mainly from the Medicaid program (American Health Care Association, 1987). In 1987, the average out of pocket expenses for a nursing home resident who required no hospitalization was $21,000 a year; the government expense accounted for, on average, another $18,730, provided of course that the resident did not require hospitalization during the year (Myers, 1987). For residents of congregate housing in Rhode Island, costs ranged from $11,940 to $19,200 annually for persons requiring personal care services, with entry fees ranging from $70,000 to $125,000 (Rhode Island Hospital, 1987). The supportive service program in place in the twelve pilot developments had an average cost of $501.18 per resident per year for the supportive services. In addition, the apartment units had section 8 rent subsidies which averaged $6,651 per year. The program is certainly the most cost effective model studied to date as well as considerably beneficial to the residents' quality of life. While independent living facilities with supportive services may not provide a level of assistance appropriate for all, it is certainly a successful model for a number of frail elderly and mentally ill residents.

REFERENCES

American Health Care Associations. (1987). Paper presented at Laventhol and Horwath Retirement Housing Conference, June 18-19, 1987.

Blazer, D.G. (1980). The epidemiology of mental illness in late life. In E.W. Busse & D.G. Blazer (Eds.), *Handbook of Geriatric Psychiatry.* New York: Van Nostrand Reinhold, pp. 249-271.

Butler, R.N. (1975). Psychiatry and the elderly: An overview. *American Journal of Psychiatry*, 132, p. 893.

Carlin, V.F. & Mansberg, R (1984). *If I Live to Be 100 . . . Congregate Housing for Later Life.* West Nyack, NY: Parker Publishing.

Cheah, K.C. (1978). The depressed elderly patient: Part I. Diagnosis and classification. *Journal of the Arkansas Medical Society*, 75, pp. 141-47.

Cohen, G.D. (1980). Prospects for mental health and aging. In J.E. Birren & R.B. Sloane (Eds.), *Handbook of Mental Health and Aging.* Englewood Cliffs, New Jersey: Prentice Hall, pp. 971-993.

Cohen, G.D. (1977). Approach to the geriatric patient. *Medical Clinics of North America*, 61, pp. 855-866.

D'Arcy, C. (1987). Aging and mental health. In V. Marshall (Ed.), *Aging in Canada: Social Perspective.* 2nd edition. Markham, Ontario: Fitzhenry & Whiteside, pp. 424-450.

Gallagher, D., Thompson, L.W., & Levy, S.M. (1980). Clinical psychological assessment of older adults. In L. Poon (Ed.), *Aging in the 1980's: Selected Contempo-*

rary Issues in the Psychology of Aging. Washington, DC: American Psychological Association.

George, L.K. (1979). The happiness syndrome: Methodological and substantive issues in the study of social psychological well-being in adulthood. *The Gerontologist*, 19, pp. 210-216.

George, L.K. &. Bearon, B. (1980). *Quality of Life in Older Persons: Meaning and Measurement.* New York: Human Sciences Press.

George, L.K. et al. (1988). Psychiatric disorders and mental health service use in later life: Evidence from the epidemiologic catchment area program. In J.A. Brody & G.L. Maddox (Eds.), *Epidemiology and Aging: An International Perspective.* New York: Springer Publishing.

Goga, J.A. & Hambacher, W.O. (1977). Psychologic and behavioral assessment of geriatric patients: A review. *Journal of American Geriatric Society*, 25, pp. 232-237.

Graney, M.J. & Graney, E.E. (1973). Scaling adjustment in older people. *International Journal on Aging and Human Development*, 4, pp. 351-359.

Heumann, L. & Boldy, D. (1982). *Housing for the Elderly: Planning and Policy Formulation in Western Europe and North America.* London: Croom Helm.

Jaco, E.G. (1960). Depression in the elderly. *Journal of the American Geriatrics Society*, 27, pp. 38-42.

Kane, R.A. & Kane, R.L. (1981). *Assessing the Elderly.* Santa Monica, CA: The Rand Corporation.

Katz, S., Hedrick, S. & Henderson, N. (1979). The measurement of long-term care needs and impact. *Health and Medical Services Review*, 2, pp. 2-21.

Kay, D.W.K. & Bergmann, K. (1980). Epidemiology of mental disorders among the aged in the community. In J.E. Birren and R.B. Sloane (Eds.), *Handbook of Mental Health and Aging.* New Jersey: Prentice Hall. pp. 34-56.

Larson, R. (1978). Thirty years of research on the subjective well-being of older Americans. *Journal of Gerontology*, 33, pp. 109-125.

Lester, D. (1994). Suicide in the elderly: An overview. In D. Lester & M. Tallmer (Eds.), *Now I Lay Me Down: Suicide in the Elderly.* Philadelphia: The Charles Press.

Marshall, V.W. (1987). *Aging in Canada: Social Perspective.* 2nd edition. Markham, Ontario: Fitzhenry & Whiteside.

Monk, A. & Kaye, L.W. (1991). Congregate housing for the elderly: Its need, function and perspectives. *Journal of Housing for the Elderly*, 9, 1/2, pp. 5-19.

Myers, A.D. (1987). A consumer view of limiting factors. Provider American Health Care Association.

National Association of Housing and Redevelopment Officials. (1985). *Monitor*, 7, p. 12.

Neugebauer, R., Dohrenwend, B.P., & Dohrenwend, B.S. (1980). Formulation of hypotheses about the true prevalence of functional psychiatric disorders among the elderly in the United States. In B.P. Dohrenwend, B.S. Dohrenwend, M.S. Gould, B. Link, R. Neugebauer, & R. Wunsch-Hitzig (Eds.), *Mental Illness in the United States: Epidemiological Estimates.* New York: Praeger.

O'Neal, P., Robins, E. & Schmidt, E.H. (1966). Psychiatric study of attempted suicide in persons over 60 years of age. *Arch. Neurol. Psychiatry*, 75, pp. 275-284.

Osgood, N.J., Brant, B.A., & Lipman, A. (1991). *Suicide Among the Elderly in Long-Term Care Facilities.* Westport, CT: Greenwood.

Raskin, A. &. Jarvik, L.F. (1979). *Psychiatric Symptoms and Cognitive Loss in the Elderly: Evaluation and Assessment Techniques.* Washington, DC: Hemisphere Publishing Company.

Rhode Island Division of Planning. (1992). Rhode Island population projections, 1995-2020. *Monthly Progress Report*, January, 1992.

Rhode Island Division of Planning. (1993). A century of population change. *Monthly Progress Report*, January, 1993.

Rhode Island Hospital. (1987). Planning study for proposed senior living community. *R.I. Hospital*, August, 1987.

Salzman, C. et al., (1972a). Rating scales for psychotropic drug research with geriatric patients: I. Behavior ratings. *Journal of the American Geriatric Society*, 20, pp. 209-214.

Salzman, C. et al. (1972b). Rating scales for psychotropic drug research with geriatric patients: II. Mood ratings. *Journal of the American Geriatric Society*, 20, pp. 215-221.

Silverman, P. (1987). *The Elderly as Modern Pioneers.* Bloomington: Indiana University Press.

U.S. Bureau of the Census. (1993). *Statistical Abstract of the United States.* Washington, DC: U.S. Department of Commerce.

World Health Organization. (1959). Mental health problems of the aging and the *aged. WHO Technical Report Series.* 171.

Differences in the Quality of Housing Units Occupied by Elderly Men versus Elderly Women

Namkee G. Choi

SUMMARY. Unmet housing needs can be more costly and more hazardous to health and well-being in the case of elderly than in the case of nonelderly, because the elderly in general spend more time in their homes. The purpose of this paper, based on the data from the 1991 wave of the American Housing Survey, is to examine the adequacy/quality of housing units headed by those aged 65 years or older and to examine factors that would predict poor-quality housing headed by older persons. The findings indicate that housing units occupied by older minority women, especially those living with relatives or with nonrelatives were the most likely to be deficient, whereas those occupied by white older women living alone were the least likely to be deficient. Policy and social service implications of the findings are also discussed. *[Article copies available for a fee from The Haworth Document Delivery Service: 1-800-342-9678. E-mail address: getinfo@haworthpressinc.com]*

KEYWORDS. Unmet housing needs, health and housing, substandard housing, elderly minority women, elderly Caucasian women

Every human being is entitled to affordable, quality housing in order to have a decent standard of living. Especially for many elderly,

Namkee G. Choi, DSW, is Associate Professor, School of Social Work, 359 Baldy Hall, SUNY at Buffalo, Buffalo, NY 14260.

[Haworth co-indexing entry note]: "Differences in the Quality of Housing Units Occupied by Elderly Men versus Elderly Women." Choi, Namkee G. Co-published simultaneously in *Journal of Housing for the Elderly* (The Haworth Press, Inc.) Vol. 13, No. 1/2, 1999, pp. 93-113; and: *Making Aging in Place Work* (ed: Leon A. Pastalan) The Haworth Press, Inc., 1999, pp. 93-113. Single or multiple copies of this article are available for a fee from The Haworth Document Delivery Service [1-800-342-9678, 9:00 a.m. - 5:00 p.m. (EST). E-mail address: getinfo@haworthpressinc.com].

93

deteriorating health and the onset of disability tie their ability to function even more closely to their housing–the primary environmental setting for them. After retirement, the elderly in general spend more time in their homes, entertaining family or friends and/or receiving care and assistance at home, than do the nonelderly. And for most elderly, an owned home is their single greatest asset. With the exception of some postretirement amenity seekers and older movers who relocate closer to kith and kin, the elderly are less likely to move and more likely to stay put than the nonelderly. The elderly have also indicated an increasing desire to "age in place" over the past several years (American Association of Retired Persons [AARP], 1994; Leather & Mackintosh, 1993). Thus, a house for an older person often becomes his/her locus of social interaction as well as independent living, with residential well-being directly related to his/her physical, financial, social, and psychological well-being (Lawton, 1989). Safe, convenient, sanitary housing units are essential if older persons are to live independently as long as possible.

With respect also to large-scale economies, the increasing numbers of the elderly require more attention to the supply, affordability, and appropriateness of their housing so as to curb the escalating cost of constructing nursing homes and placing people in them. Currently, nearly a quarter of all U.S. households are headed by persons aged 65 years or older. With the increasing proportion of elderly in the population, the number of households headed by them–especially single-person and very old households–will certainly increase in the future, creating an expanded need for housing assistance (Katsura, Struyk, & Newman, 1989). The shelter needs and housing conditions of these households should be priority concerns of aging policy and services.

To date, however, housing for the elderly has not had as high a priority as their income security and health care. Although the quality of housing units occupied by older persons has not been found to be different from the quality of housing units occupied by nonelderly persons (Golant & LaGreca, 1995), unmet housing needs can certainly be more costly and more hazardous to health and well-being in the case of elderly than in the case of nonelderly, for reasons mentioned above.

The purpose of this paper is to examine the adequacy/quality of housing units headed by those aged 65 years or older and to examine factors that would predict poor-quality housing headed by older persons. The primary focus will be, first, on the comparison of units headed by older women with those headed by older men, and, second, on the association of gender, minority status, and living arrangements with housing quality. Because minority elderly are more likely to be poor than are white elderly, they are more likely to live in inadequate housing units. And because single, older minority women who live alone, with relatives (other than spouses), or with nonrelatives are especially more likely to be poor than are older men and women, of both majority and minority, who live with spouses, they are also more likely to live in inadequate housing units. Policy and social service implications of the findings will also be discussed.

LITERATURE REVIEW

The quality of housing environment is a key determinant of older persons' quality of life, because they spend a large share of time–as much as 80 to 90 percent of their lives–at home (Cox, 1993; Struyk & Katsura, 1987). As a person ages, a house increasingly becomes a place of identity, a symbol of one's status in the community, and a "manifestation of one's power to choose, to exercise autonomy" (Tilson & Fahey, 1990, p. xv). The "significance of 'home' increases as older persons face the loss of other symbols of independence and connections to the mainstream of life" (Sykes, 1990, p. 53). And the two most powerful predictors of well-being among the elderly are their perceived health and housing satisfaction (Berresi, Ferraro, & Hobey, 1983-1984). This is apparently so, even though the elderly tend to underestimate the seriousness of their housing problems (Golant, 1992; Leather & Mackintosh, 1993).

With the progression of aging and the onset of physical and functional disabilities, housing is often a factor determining whether an older person remains in the community or not, because housing conditions can have a dramatic effect on a chronically ill or disabled person's ability to function and perform everyday activities (Struyk & Katsura, 1987). Moreover, certain housing characteristics have been found to be correlated with a family's willingness to care for an elderly relative and to be essential to reducing demands on caregivers and to enable them to effectively provide caregiving (AARP, 1994; Newman, 1985; Struyk & Katsura, 1987). Even for the well elderly, poor housing conditions may be a potential cause of diminished social support for them, because they may not want to entertain family or friends at home due to embarrassment about their housing conditions (Maguire, 1991). Thus, in lieu of person-environment transactions, housing as a physical environment poses as decisive opportunities as well as constraints on the elderly's performance of their daily lives and on their physical and psychological well-being (Golant, 1984; Lawton, 1989).

But housing situations in later life often mirror the economic status of older persons. The elderly in general have the highest rate of home-ownership of all age groups. But older renters tend to be poorer than younger renters and to consist of minority group members and very old women (Redfoot & Gaberlavage, 1991). In terms also of the housing quality of the elderly, previous studies have found that black elderly households, both owners and renters, and to a lesser extent Hispanic elderly households, were in worse-quality housing than white elderly households (Golant & LaGreca, 1994a). Also, elderly households in nonmetropolitan rural areas and in rural parts of metro-politan areas had the highest housing-deficiency rates in the country. Within metropolitan areas, central cities had the worst-quality housing stocks, and the urban suburbs had the lowest rate of physical deficien-cy (Golant & LaGreca, 1994b). Given the lifelong economic disad-vantage and deprivation of minorities as well as the bleak economic situations of many residents of central cities and rural areas, these findings are not surprising. Income is a significant predictor of the likelihood of any one-time as well as sustained home repair and main-tenance—heating, electrical, plumbing, interior and exterior—among el-derly homeowners (Reschovsky & Newman, 1990; Struyk & Katsura, 1987). Apparently, the elderly who have had economic resources could afford the sustained repair and improvement required to enjoy a better housing environment.

With the aging process, gaps between the poor and the nonpoor, the healthy and the disabled, and the socially well-integrated and the socially isolated are often magnified. Despite the income-equalizing effects of social security, other sources of retirement income such as private pensions and asset income further polarize the income gap among the elderly (Crystal & Shea, 1990). Because income is posi-tively associated with health and social integration, the poor minority elderly and elderly women are also more likely to suffer from poor health and social isolation than are the well-off elderly and elderly men (Ferraro, 1987; Herzog, 1989). Especially women "not only enter old age poorer than men but become poorer with age as a consequence of widowhood, higher health care expenditures, and pay and pension inequities" (Minkler & Stone, 1985, p. 353). Needless to say, the situation is worse for women who are members of ethnic minority groups and women who live alone (Gonyea, 1994; Minkler & Stone, 1985).

Considering their longer life expectancy, lower economic status, and poorer health, single older women, as compared to their married counterparts and to older men, are more likely to live in physically deficient housing units and to have greater needs for housing assistance. But few previous studies analyzed differences in the housing quality of the elderly by gender and living arrangement. With increasing numbers of single female heads of households, future elderly households will consist of a larger proportion of elderly women who are poor and living alone. Although many white older women who live alone tend to do so because they can afford to (Choi, 1991), many of their baby boom generation counterparts may not have any choice but to live alone in their old age, regardless of what they can afford, because they do not have children or they have fewer children than their predecessors. As for black and Hispanic older women, regardless of their living arrangements, their economic status has been and will continue to be a barrier to their affording decent housing or keeping their houses in decent shape. Moreover, poor minority older women are the most likely of all elderly persons to be trapped in neighborhoods that are infested with crime and violence and/or that have limited access to social services and public transportation.

Current social policies and programs to assist the elderly with their housing needs are limited to public housing units and rent subsidy programs–Sections 8 and 202, primarily. The only program specifically focused on helping elderly homeowners keep up their housing units to increase their freedom of movement is the Farmers Home Administration (FHA) Section 504 grant program. Although other sources of funding for housing rehabilitation include the Community Development Block Grant (CDBG) and Title III of the Older Americans Act (OAA), the funding through these sources has to compete with many other programs. Moreover, since none of these programs is flexible enough to address both substandard housing conditions and adaptations needed to promote mobility, poor minority elderly are underserved by them (Redfoot & Gaberlavage, 1991). The National Affordable Housing Act of 1990 expanded the FHA home equity conversion demonstration program, which allows older homeowners to use their home equity to meet home repair needs. But the program has yet to reach many older persons. In order to preserve and enhance older persons' autonomy and independence, their housing problems need to be identified and remedied. Especially for poor older women, decent living environments that foster their independence, dignity, and social integration are essential if they are to carry on a healthy and dignified life in their old age.

SAMPLE AND DATA

The source of data for this study is the 1991 wave of the American Housing Survey (AHS): National File, a longitudinal survey that started in 1973 and was funded and managed by the Department of Housing and Urban Development (HUD) and produced by the U.S. Bureau of the Census. The total sample size of the 1991 AHS is 44,764 housing units (i.e., after excluding vacant units that were in the sample), representing a universe of more than 90 million housing units in the United States (Hadden & Leger, 1990). Because housing units, not persons, are the units of analysis, the findings from the AHS are generalizable to households or dwelling units as opposed to individuals.

Of 44,764 sample housing units, 10,285 units, or 23%, were occupied by age 65 and older household heads, or "reference persons," who owned or rented the units. The elderly household heads in this analysis are defined as those aged 65 and older because a majority of people retire between ages 60 and 65. The economic status and residential circumstances often undergo changes with retirement, and the analysis in this paper attempts to capture postretirement housing conditions of the elderly. Of 10,285 sample units headed by older persons, 3,702 units contained at least one additional elderly member, with 3,315 units containing elderly spouse of the head. Of 34,479 sample units headed by nonelderly persons (those under age 65), 887 units contained at least one elderly relative of the head. For the analysis in this paper, however, only housing units headed by elderly persons were included because detailed information is often not available for those who are not heads.

As shown in Table 1, 54.0% of the elderly household heads were

TABLE 1. Gender Differences in Sociodemographic and Economic Characteristics of Elderly Household Heads

	Male	Female
n	5,549	4,736
Age (Years)		
65-74	64.8%	47.7%
75-84	29.5	40.1
85+	5.8	12.2
Race		
White	88.0%	85.1%
Black	7.4	10.9
Hispanic	3.0	3.1
Other	1.6	0.9
Marital status		
Married	76.6%	6.1%
Widowed	13.5	76.1
Divorced	4.7	9.6
Separated	1.3	1.8
Never-married	4.0	6.3
Living arrangements		
With a spouse	75.5%	5.2%
Alone	17.6	74.5
With an unmarried child	2.3	12.6
With a parent	0	0.5
With a sibling	0.6	2.3
With other relatives	2.9	3.0
With nonrelatives	1.1	1.9
Median annual household income	$20,000	$10,300
Poverty status		
Below 100% of the OPL[a]	9.8%	25.8%
Below 125% of the OPL	17.1%	39.5%
Housing tenure		
Own/buying	85.3%	68.0%
Rent	13.2	28.9
Rent for free	1.5	3.1
Region of residence		
Northeast	21.0%	23.4%
Midwest	24.5	25.7
South	35.0	33.5
West	19.4	17.4

TABLE 1 (continued)

n	Male 5,549	Female 4,736
Central city/suburban status		
Central city	27.5%	33.4%
Urban/urbanized suburb	32.3	31.1
Rural, nonmetro	17.6	14.0
Rural suburb	13.1	9.2
Urban, nonmetro	9.6	12.4
Median monthly housing cost	$258	$230
Median housing cost share of income	15.8%	25.5%
Median length of occupancy (years)	21.0	19.0
Percentage without own means of transportation	7.7%	35.1%

[a]Official poverty line
Note: Statistics are all weighted.

male and 46.0% female. A higher proportion of the female than the male household heads were black. As expected, there were significant gender differences in the marital status and age distribution: 76.6% of the elderly male household heads, as compared to only 6.1% of the elderly female household heads, were married, and women were twice as likely to be 85 years and older as were men. Nearly three-fourths of the units headed by women, as opposed to less than one-fifth of the units headed by men, were occupied by only the household head. The elderly female household heads were also more likely to have their children living with them than were the elderly male household heads. (Because the older persons were household heads, it is more likely that the relatives moved in with the older persons than vice versa.) As also expected, the households headed by women were poorer and less likely to be owner-occupied units than were those headed by men. The women were also less likely to own means of transportation than were the men.

MEASURES AND METHODS

The quality of housing is measured by the HUD measure of housing inadequacy: Adequate, moderately deficient, and severely deficient. A housing unit is considered *severely deficient* (or *severely inadequate*) if it has any of the following five problems:

Plumbing: Lacking hot piped water or a flush toilet, or lacking both bathtub and shower, all for the exclusive use of the unit.

Heating: Having been uncomfortably cold in the preceding winter, for 24 hours or more, because the heating equipment broke down, with the equipment having broken down at least three times in the preceding winter, for at least six hours each time.

Upkeep: Having any five of the following six maintenance problems in the preceding 90 days: leaks from outdoors; leaks from indoors; holes in the floor; holes or open cracks in the walls or ceilings; more than a square foot of peeling paint or plaster; or rats.

Hallways: Having all of the following four problems in public areas: no working light fixtures; loose or missing steps; loose or missing railings; and no elevator.

Electric: Having no electricity, or all of the following three electrical problems; exposed wiring; a room with no working wall outlet; and three blown fuses or tripped circuit breakers in the preceding 90 days.

A housing unit is considered *moderately deficient* (or *moderately inadequate*) if it has any of the following five problems, but none of the severe problems:

Plumbing: Having the toilets all break down at the same time, at least three times in the preceding three months, for at least six hours each time.

Heating: Having unvented gas, oil, or kerosene heaters as the main source of heat; these give off unsafe fumes.

Upkeep: Having any three of the six upkeep problems mentioned as *severely deficient* or *severely inadequate*.

Hallways: Having any three of the four hallways problems mentioned as *severely deficient* or *severely inadequate*.

Kitchen: Lacking a sink, range, or refrigerator, all for the exclusive use of the unit.

The shortcomings of the HUD measure were discussed in previous studies (Golant & LaGreca, 1994a; Golant & LaGreca, 1994b). Although these and other previous studies based on the AHS (Golant & LaGreca, 1994c; Golant & LaGreca, 1995) also used a composite numerical measure of housing quality, this study uses the HUD measure only because it was strongly positively correlated with the numerical measure.

Descriptive bivariate relationships between housing quality and a variety of variables are presented. But, because of the large sample size, statistical tests of significance–especially in the case of a small-percentage-point difference between cells–tend to be exaggerated and thus are not included. Following descriptive statistics, two maximum likelihood logit regression models were adopted to analyze the determinants of housing quality. The dependent variable, housing quality, is given the value of 1 if the HUD measure indicated that the unit was moderately or severely deficient and the value of 0 if the HUD measure indicated that the unit was *not* moderately or severely deficient (thus, adequate). Because the overall risk of housing deficiency was so small (7.8% of all housing units), the maximum likelihood estimates of coefficients were obtained by taking a 10% random sample of adequate units but including 100% of all inadequate units of the original HUD sample. Logit regression models are known to be flexible enough to take such data without a need for further differential weighing and corrections for degrees of freedom (Gortmaker, 1979).

Model I analyzes the independent effects of gender (female, 1; male, 0), race (White, 1; Black, 2; Hispanic, 3), and living arrangements (lived with spouse, 1; lived alone, 2; lived with other relatives or nonrelatives, 3) of the heads as determinants of housing quality, controlling for the following variables: age (65 to 74 years, 1; 75 to 84 years, 2; 85 years and older, 3); level of education (in years of last grade attended); housing tenure (own, 1; rent for money or rent for free, 0); length of time lived in the housing unit (in years); total household income as percentage of poverty level (below 125% of the poverty level, 1; other, 0); percentage of household income used for housing cost, including mortgage payment, real property tax, rent, and utilities, (higher than 33%, 1; 33% or lower, 0); region (Northeast, 1; Midwest, 2; South, 3; West, 4), and central city/suburban status (central city/additional central city, 1; urban/urbanized suburb, 2; rural, nonmetropolitan, 3; rural suburbs, 4; urban/urbanized area, nonmetropolitan, 5). With respect to living arrangements, those who lived with relatives other than spouses and those who lived with nonrelatives were collapsed together, because the two groups were similar in housing deficiency rate. Marital status was not included because of its multicolinearity with type of living arrangement.

Model II analyzes the compounded effects of sex, race, and living arrangements in a more explicit way (i.e., what is the likelihood that severely or moderately deficient housing units will be occupied by each of the following groups rather than by white male household heads who had other relatives or nonrelatives living with them?): white females who lived with spouses, 1; white females who lived alone, 2; white females who had other relatives or nonrelatives living with them, 3; black or Hispanic females who lived with spouses, 4; black or Hispanic females who lived alone, 5; black or Hispanic females who had other relatives or nonrelatives living with them, 6; white males who lived with spouses, 7; white males who lived alone, 8; black or Hispanic males who lived with spouses, 9; black or Hispanic males who lived alone, 10; black or Hispanic males who had other relatives or nonrelatives living with them, 11. The covariates for Model II are the same as those for Model I. Because of the small sample size, racial categories other than white, black (including black Hispanics), and Hispanics were excluded from these multivariate analyses.

FINDINGS

Bivariate analysis: As shown in Table 2, 8.8% of housing units occupied by elderly women and 6.9% of those occupied by elderly men were moderately or severely deficient according to the HUD standard. No significant gender difference was found in terms also of the elderly household heads' satisfaction with their housing units and their neighborhoods. The mean satisfaction scores suggest that the elderly are in general very satisfied with their residential environments. But both men and women living in deficient units had significantly lower satisfaction with their residential environments than did those living in adequate units (see Table 3).

The quality of units occupied by the young old (65 to 74 years), the middle old (75 to 84 years), and the old old (85 years and older) was not different. The difference in quality between owned and rented (with money) units does not appear to be significant, either. But the units rented free of charge (which consist of only 2.2% of the units occupied by the elderly) appear to have a high deficiency rate. The data also show that adequate units and severely deficient units were not different in terms of length of time (years) elderly household heads

TABLE 2. Differences in Quality of Housing Units Headed by Older Men and Women (%)

	n	Adequate	Moderately deficient	Severely deficient
All	(10,285)	92.3	4.8	3.0
Sex				
Men	(5,549)	93.1	4.1	2.8
Women	(4,736)	91.3	5.6	3.2
Age (years)				
65-74	(5,853)	92.6	4.7	2.7
75-84	(3,535)	92.0	4.6	3.3
85+	(897)	91.1	5.8	3.1
Race				
White	(8,912)	94.0	3.3	2.7
Black	(930)	78.0	17.2	4.8
Hispanic	(314)	85.5	10.3	4.3
Other	(129)	93.3	1.0	5.6
Housing tenure				
Own/buying	(7,953)	92.9	4.4	2.8
Rent	(2,101)	91.0	5.6	3.4
Rent for free	(231)	82.9	10.9	6.1
Region				
Northeast	(2,273)	95.2	2.2	2.6
Midwest	(2,580)	96.1	1.5	2.4
South	(3,531)	86.3	10.2	3.5
West	(1,901)	94.6	2.3	3.1
Central city/suburban status				
Central city	(3,106)	91.7	5.3	2.9
Urban(ized) suburb	(3,262)	95.8	2.0	2.2
Rural, non-metro	(1,640)	88.4	7.3	4.3
Rural, suburb	(1,162)	91.6	5.3	3.1
Urban, non-metro	(1,116)	89.5	7.2	3.2
Living arrangement				
With a spouse	(4,434)	94.5	3.3	2.2
Alone	(4,501)	91.4	5.4	3.2
With relatives	(1,195)	88.0	7.3	4.7
With nonrelatives	(155)	87.4	7.7	4.9
Living arrangement × sex				
Men living with spouses	(4,189)	94.6	3.3	2.1

	n	Adequate	Moderately deficient	Severely deficient
Living arrangement × sex (continued)				
Men living alone	(974)	88.2	7.0	4.7
Men living with relatives or with nonrelatives	(386)	88.8	5.7	5.5
Women living with spouses	(245)	92.3	4.1	3.6
Women living alone	(3,526)	92.2	5.0	2.8
Women living with relatives or with nonrelatives	(964)	87.6	8.0	4.4
Race × sex				
White men	(4,884)	94.2	3.2	2.6
White women	(4,028)	93.7	3.6	2.8
Black men	(412)	81.0	15.1	4.0
Black women	(518)	75.6	18.9	5.5
Hispanic men	(168)	89.1	7.5	3.5
Hispanic women	(146)	81.3	13.5	5.2
Other men	(86)	94.6	0	5.4
Other women	(43)	90.8	3.1	6.1
Race × sex × living arrangement[a]				
White women living with spouses	(198)	94.5	3.0	2.4
White women living alone	(3,095)	94.0	3.5	2.6
White women living with relatives	(735)	92.1	4.2	3.7
Black/Hispanic women living with spouses	(42)	80.9	9.3	9.8
Black/Hispanic women living alone	(404)	79.0	16.7	4.3
Black/Hispanic women living with relatives	(218)	72.1	21.2	6.7
White men living with spouses	(3,779)	95.5	2.5	2.0
White men living alone	(793)	89.9	5.6	4.6
White men living with relatives	(312)	89.9	4.7	5.5
Black/Hispanic men living with spouses	(342)	84.5	12.5	3.1
Black/Hispanic men living alone	(171)	80.3	14.4	5.3
Black/Hispanic men living with relatives	(67)	85.2	11.0	3.8

[a]Because of a small sample size, "other" races were excluded.

TABLE 3. Gender Difference in Household Heads' Satisfaction with Their Housing Units and Neighborhood: On a Scale of 1 (Worst) to 10 (Best)

	Men	Women
n	5,549	4,736
Satisfaction with housing		
Mean (SD)	8.71 (1.66)	8.70 (1.70)
Satisfaction with neighborhood		
Mean (SD)	8.35 (2.15)	8.40 (2.16)
Housing quality × satisfaction with housing		
Adequate: Mean (SD)	8.78 (1.58)	8.78 (1.60)
Moderately deficient: Mean (SD)	7.59 (2.31)	7.93 (2.30)
Severely deficient: Mean (SD)	7.96 (2.34)	7.77 (2.52)
Housing quality × satisfaction with neighborhood		
Adequate: Mean (SD)	8.40 (2.10)	8.45 (2.08)
Moderately deficient: Mean (SD)	7.64 (2.73)	7.78 (2.88)
Severely deficient: Mean (SD)	7.70 (2.62)	7.99 (2.75)

Note: For both men and women, those who lived in moderately or severely deficient units had significantly lower housing and neighborhood scores than did those who lived in adequate units (p < .05).

lived in them. But moderately deficient units were occupied by heads significantly longer than the other units. In terms of regional difference, housing quality in the South appears to be much lower than in the other regions. Also, housing quality in rural and urban nonmetropolitan areas appears to be lower than in urban suburbs.

An interesting finding was related to living arrangements. The quality of housing occupied by the elderly whose relatives or nonrelatives lived with them was more likely to be deficient than was housing occupied by the elderly who lived with spouses or lived alone. When household heads were separated by gender, however, an interesting and marked difference appeared. The units occupied by elderly men who lived alone were almost twice as likely to be deficient as those occupied by elderly men who lived with their spouses. On the other hand, the quality of units occupied by elderly women who lived alone was not different from that of units occupied by elderly women who lived with their spouses, and they were much less likely to be deficient than the units occupied by elderly women who lived with other relatives or with nonrelatives.

But the most marked finding was the racial difference: 22.0% of housing units occupied by black household heads and 14.6% of those occupied by Hispanic household heads were deficient as opposed to 6.0% of those occupied by whites. Most notably, 25% of housing units occupied by black women and 18.7% of those occupied by Hispanic women, as compared to 6.4% of those occupied by white women, were deficient. The units occupied by black or Hispanic men are also much more likely to be deficient than those occupied by white men or white women.

Multivariate analysis: As shown in Table 4, the results of Model I confirm the results of bivariate analyses. The maximum likelihood logit regression coefficients indicate that age and sex in themselves were not significant predictors of housing deficiency. Housing units occupied by white household heads were significantly less likely but those occupied by black household heads were significantly more likely to be deficient than those occupied by Hispanic household heads. Units occupied by older couples were less likely to be deficient than those occupied by older persons who lived with other relatives or with nonrelatives. Those occupied by older persons who lived alone were not different from the latter. Units occupied by persons with higher education and by owners, as opposed to renters, were less likely to be deficient. On the other hand, the units occupied by the same persons for a longer period of time and by persons whose household income was below 125% of the official poverty threshold were more likely to be deficient. When the poverty status and other covariates were controlled, the sign of the coefficient for the percentage of income spent on housing was also positive. That is, other things being equal, those who spent less than 34% of their income for housing were more likely to reside in deficient units than were those who spent 34% or more of their income for housing. Housing units located in the Midwest were less likely but those located in the South were more likely to be deficient than those located in the West. Housing units located in urban suburbs were less likely but units located in rural, nonmetropolitan areas were more likely to be deficient than units in urban, nonmetropolitan areas. The quality of housing units in central cities and rural suburbs was not different from that of units in urban, nonmetropolitan areas.

As for the compounded effects of gender, race, and living arrangements, the results of Model II show that units occupied by white

TABLE 4. Logistic Regression Coefficients of Determinants of Housing Quality

	Model I B (SE)	Model II B (SE)
Sex (Male)	−.271 (.145)	
Race		
White	−.465 (.115)**	
Black	.322 (.131)*	
Living arrangement		
With a spouse	−.337 (.105)**	
Alone	−.003 (.087)	
Age		
65-74	.160 (.086)	.152 (.087)
75-84	.001 (.087)	.018 (.088)
Years of education	−.040 (.016)*	−.040 (.017)*
Housing tenure (own/buying)	−.600 (.147)**	−.588 (.147)**
Years of occupancy	.019 (.004)**	.020 (.004)**
Poverty status (below 125% of OPL)	.505 (.136)**	.559 (.138)**
Share of housing cost of income		
(less than 34%)	.508 (.136)**	.516 (.137)**
Region		
Northeast	−.173 (.111)	−.185 (.112)
Midwest	−.593 (.104)**	−.585 (.105)**
South	.647 (.086)**	.660 (.087)**
Central city/suburban status		
Central city	−.118 (.098)	−.124 (.099)
Urban suburb	−.393 (.106)**	−.387 (.107)**
Rural, nonmetro	.305 (.114)*	.295 (.115)*
Rural, suburb	−.060 (.133)	−.062 (.134)
Race × sex × living arrangement		
White women living with spouses		−.184 (.413)
White women living alone		−.668 (.146)**
White women living with relatives		−.315 (.210)
Black/Hispanic women living with spouses		.942 (.770)
Black/Hispanic women living alone		−.118 (.213)
Black/Hispanic women living with relatives		1.024 (.298)**
White men living with spouses		−.757 (.149)**
White men living alone		.038 (.194)
Black/Hispanic men living with spouses		.257 (.262)
Black/Hispanic men living alone		.289 (.332)
Black/Hispanic men living with relatives		−.431 (.473)
−2LL Model Chi-square (df)	355.35 (19)**	377.86 (25)**

women living alone and white men living with wives were significantly less likely to be deficient than were units occupied by white men living with relatives or with nonrelatives. But units occupied by black or Hispanic women who lived with relatives or with nonrelatives were significantly more likely to be deficient than were units occupied by the latter. (Further analysis showed that the average income of white women who lived alone was almost twice the average per capita income of black or Hispanic women household heads who lived with relatives/nonrelatives [$12,977 vs. $7,480, p < .01]. The average income of white men who lived with relatives/nonrelatives, $13,442, was not statistically different from the average income of white women who lived alone but was significantly less than the average per capita income of white men who lived with their spouses.)

DISCUSSION AND IMPLICATIONS

The above analysis confirmed the findings of previous studies that housing tenure, region, location, race, and income are associated with the quality of housing occupied by elderly persons. In addition, this study found that, other things being equal, both length of residential occupancy and percentage of income spent on housing are positively correlated with the likelihood of housing deficiency. Living arrangement is also an important predictor of housing deficiency. As expected, units occupied by elderly couples were less likely to be deficient than those occupied by older persons living alone, or living with relatives or nonrelatives.

But, most important of all, this analysis indicates that housing units occupied by older minority women, especially those living with relatives or with nonrelatives, were the most likely to be deficient, whereas those occupied by white older women living alone were the least likely to be deficient. Thus, racial differences within the female gender appear to be more serious than gender differences per se. The living arrangements are important because, in the case of white older women, they often reflect the women's economic status. As mentioned earlier, white older women who live alone tend to do so because they can afford independent living. But the living arrangements of minority older women do not appear to be associated with affordability, because the average per capita income of minority women did not differ by living arrangement.

Given that all minority women were equally likely to be poor, it is not clear why the housing units occupied by older minority women who lived with relatives or with nonrelatives, as compared to those occupied by older minority women who lived with spouses or alone, were especially likely to be deficient. It may be that their poor health was the reason for their coresidence with relatives or nonrelatives and for the lack of upkeep of their housing units. Unfortunately, however, the AHS data do not include any information on health status of household heads. Another speculation is based on the findings of previous studies (Aquilino, 1990; Gratton, 1987). That is, minority elderly parents are more likely than white elderly parents to take in and support their adult children or other relatives when the latter have a tough time making it. If so, some minority elderly parents who coreside with their children/relatives are in fact likely to be heavily burdened economically.

With increasing numbers of single older women, especially single older minority women, the quality of their housing needs special attention. Their inferior economic and health statuses make it very important for them to have adequate housing that can facilitate, not debilitate their daily functioning. Nevertheless, the housing situation of these single minority women is not given any special attention.

Although housing units occupied by minority older men, both married and single, may be a little less likely to be deficient than those occupied by their female counterparts, they are still more likely to be deficient than are units occupied by whites of both sexes. Such racial difference is primarily due to differences in the economic status of the two groups. The housing situations of minority older men also needs special attention.

Based on these findings, the following policy and social service measures are recommended. First, the severe housing needs, along with economic, health, social service needs of single minority women must be recognized. Oftentimes, social services focus on older persons who live alone, while those who live with relatives are, as in the case of SSI, penalized because of the assumption that the relatives are supporting them. But the findings of this study show that minority women who live with relatives or with nonrelatives may be in a more needy situation than those who live alone.

Second, given that minority older persons in general face a high risk of housing deficiency, and that housing deficiency is highly correlated with poverty status and housing tenure, it is necessary for social service providers to check the adequacy of their clients' housing, especially if they are poor renters. A checklist for housing adequacy needs to be incorporated as an essential long-term care assessment tool for this population.

Third, once the needs are recognized and identified, it is necessary that housing support systems for older persons be instituted or improved. Existing public housing and rent subsidy programs need to be expanded because they invariably have long waiting lists. Funding for new construction of low-income housing such as provided in the Section 202 program needs to be improved. Without major increases in public expenditure for low-income housing, poor renters (both elderly and nonelderly) will continue to face difficulty finding decent, affordable housing units.

Fourth, because a majority of the elderly are homeowners who prefer to age in place, a system that provides advice and that supports, financially or otherwise, small home repair and maintenance functions of elderly homeowners themselves is another option. For older persons whose units need more extensive rehabilitation or professional assistance, HUD and social service agencies need to collaborate to institute a system of such assistance. Rehabilitation of deficient housing and remodeling of housing in lieu of changing residential environmental needs of older persons will certainly save taxpayers money in the long run because it will prevent premature institutionalization. The FHA Section 504 grant program needs increased funding to truly serve those who need it. Also, funding for housing rehabilitation needs to be separated from such multipurpose block grants as CDBG and Title III of the OAA and become an independent, single-purpose block or categorical grant.

Fifth, in the face of shrinking federal subsidy for low-income housing and housing assistance, it is necessary for social service agencies to come up with creative ideas and programs to improve and adapt the housing environment of the elderly. For example, social service agencies and local HUD offices can mobilize volunteer corps who can provide housing advice and/or free labor for older persons. Self-help organizations for housing rehabilitation in the neighborhoods can also be organized. These groups may be able to arrange the purchase of building and maintenance materials at wholesale prices and supply labor and skills at no cost or lower than market cost.

REFERENCES

Aquilino, W. S. (1990). The likelihood of parent-adult child coresidence: Effects of family structure and parental characteristics. *Journal of Marriage and the Family*, 52, 405-419.

American Association of Retired Persons (1994). *Understanding senior housing for the 1990's: Survey of consumer preferences, concerns, and needs.*

Berresi, C. M., Ferraro, K. F., & Hobey, L. L. (1983-1984). Environmental satisfaction, sociability and wellbeing among urban elderly. *International Journal of Aging and Human Development*, 18, 277-284.

Choi, N. G. (1991). Racial differences in the determinants of living arrangements of widowed and divorced elderly women. *The Gerontologist*, 31, 496-504.

Cox, H. G. (1993). *Later life: The realities of aging.* Englewood Cliffs, N.J.: Prentice Hall.

Crystal, S. & Shea, D. (1990). Cumulative advantage, cumulative disadvantage, and inequality among elderly people. *The Gerontologist*, 30, 437-443.

Ferraro, K. F. (1987). Double jeopardy to health for Black older adults? *The Journals of Gerontology*, 42, 528-533.

Golant, S. M. (1992). *Housing America's elderly: Many possibilities/few choices.* Newbury Park: Sage.

Golant, S. M. (1984). The effects of residential and activity behaviors on old people's environmental experiences. In I. Altman, M. P. Lawton, & J. F. Wohlwill (Eds.). *Elderly people and the environment* (239-278). New York: Plenum Press.

Golant, S. M. & LaGreca, A. J. (1994a). Differences in the housing quality of White, Black, and Hispanic U. S. elderly households. *The Journal of Applied Gerontology*, 14, 413-347.

Golant, S. M. & LaGreca, A. J. (1994b). City-suburban, metro-nonmetro, and regional differences in the housing quality of U. S. elderly households. *Research on Aging*, 16, 322-346.

Golant, S. M. & LaGreca, A. J. (1994c). Housing quality of U.S. elderly households: Does aging in place matter? *The Gerontologist*, 34, 803-814.

Golant, S. M. & LaGreca, A. J. (1995). The relative deprivation of U.S. elderly households as judged by their housing problems. *The Journals of Gerontology*, 50B, S13-S23.

Gonyea, G. J. (1994). The paradox of the advantaged elderly and the feminization of poverty. *Social Work*, 39, 35-41.

Gortmaker, S. L. (1979). Poverty and infant mortality in the United States. *American Sociological Review*, 44, 280-297.

Gratton, B. (1987). Familism among the Black and Mexican-American elderly: Myth or reality? *Journal of Aging Studies*, 1, 19-32.

Hadden, L. & Leger, M. (1990). *Codebook for the American Housing Survey.* Cambridge, MA: Abt Associates.

Herzog, A. R. (1989). Physical and mental health in older women: Selected research issues and data sources. In A. G. Herzog, K. C. Holden, & M. M. Seltzer (Eds.). *Health and economic status of older women: Research issues and data sources.* Amityville, NY: Baywood Publishing.

Katsura, H. M., Struyk, R. J., & Newman, S. J. (1989). *Housing for the elderly in 2010.* Washington, DC: Urban Institute.

Lawton, M. P. (1989). Housing for the elderly in the mid-1980s. In G. Lesnoff-Caravaglia (Ed.). *Handbook of applied gerontology* (341-349). New York: Human Sciences Press.

Leather, P. & Mackintosh, S. (1993). The long term impact of staying put. *Ageing and Society,* 13, 193-211.

Maguire, L. (1991). *Social support systems in practice.* Silver Spring, MD: National Association of Social Workers.

Minkler, M. & Stone, R. (1985). The feminization of poverty and older women. *The Gerontologist,* 25, 351-357.

Newman, S. (1985). Housing and long-term care: The suitability of the elderly's housing to the provision of in-home services. *The Gerontologist,* 25, 35-40.

Redfoot, D. & Gaberlavage, G. (1991). Housing for older Americans: Sustaining the dream. *Generations,* 15, 35-38.

Reschovsky, J. D. & Newman, S. J. (1990). Adaptations for independent living by older frail households. *The Gerontologist,* 30, 543-552.

Struyk, R. J. & Katsura, H. M. (1987). Aging at home: How the elderly adjust their housing without moving. *Journal of Housing for the Elderly,* 4, 1-175.

Sykes, J. T. (1990). Living independently with neighbors who care: Strategies to facilitate aging in place. In D. Tilson (Ed.). *Aging in place* (53-74). Glenview, IL: Scott, Foresman and Company.

Tilson, D. & Fahey, C. J. (1990). Introduction. In D. Tilson (Ed.). *Aging in place* (xv-xxxiii). Glenview, IL: Scott, Foresman and Company.

A Case Study Evaluation
of the Homecare Suite:
A New Long-Term Care Option for Elders

Deborah E. Altus
R. Mark Mathews

SUMMARY. Four families participated in a pilot test of the Homecare Suite–a private, fully accessible, modular apartment for elders that can be temporarily installed in the garage of a family caregiver's home. Each family took part in at least two in-depth interviews before and during their use of the Homecare Suite. Results showed that the users and caregivers were satisfied with the Homecare Suite and preferred it to alternatives for reasons including increased peace of mind, ease of providing care, accessibility, privacy, and cost. This study suggests that the Homecare Suite is deserving of further study as a long-term care option. *[Article copies available for a fee from The Haworth Document Delivery Service: 1-800-342-9678. E-mail address: getinfo@haworthpressinc.com]*

Deborah E. Altus and R. Mark Mathews are both affiliated with the Gerontology Center, University of Kansas, Lawrence, KS.

Address correspondence to Deborah Altus, Gerontology Center, 4089 Dole Center, University of Kansas, Lawrence, KS 66045.

The authors would like to acknowledge Rhonda Montgomery and Karl Kosloski for their advice and assistance with this project. The Homecare Suite was designed by Stephen Menke, President, Mobile Care, Inc., 2501 10th Street, Great Bend, KS 67530.

This research was supported by the National Institute on Aging (1-R43AG11517-01) and the Kansas Department on Aging (93-01-1SURVEY). The first author was supported by a training grant from the National Institute of Child Health and Human Development (HD07173).

[Haworth co-indexing entry note]: "A Case Study Evaluation of the Homecare Suite: A New Long-Term Care Option for Elders." Altus, Deborah E., and R. Mark Mathews Co-published simultaneously in *Journal of Housing for the Elderly* (The Haworth Press, Inc.) Vol. 13, No. 1/2, 1999, pp. 115-125; and: *Making Aging in Place Work* (ed: Leon A. Pastalan) The Haworth Press, Inc., 1999, pp. 115-125. Single or multiple copies of this article are available for a fee from The Haworth Document Delivery Service [1-800-342-9678, 9:00 a.m. - 5:00 p.m. (EST). E-mail address: getinfo@haworthpressinc.com].

115

KEYWORDS. Family caregiving, elder cottage, shared housing, assisted living, accessibility

While home care is often touted as a solution to the problems of institutionalization, families wishing to care for an elderly relative at home may encounter a variety of obstacles. Maintaining good family relations becomes difficult in crowded conditions. Stairs, narrow doorways, thick carpeting and inaccessible bathroom facilities make caring for an elder with a mobility impairment difficult and dangerous. While home renovations may solve some of these problems, renovations may be expensive, time consuming and limited by zoning laws. Further, families may be reluctant to make permanent modifications to their homes for temporary use.

A new alternative that may avoid these problems is the Homecare Suite, a fully accessible modular apartment designed to be temporarily installed in an attached garage. The Homecare Suite offers the independence of a private apartment while allowing easy access to caregivers. It avoids the zoning and lot-size issues faced by Elder Cottages (see, 1988; Lazarowich, 1991) because it is erected inside an existing structure. Unlike adding an accessory apartment, the Homecare Suite can be installed in two days and does not require permanent modifications.

The purpose of this study, funded as a small business innovation grant by the National Institute on Aging, was to conduct a preliminary evaluation of the Homecare Suite. Family case studies were designed to allow for close examination of the benefits and drawbacks of using this new housing alternative.

METHOD

Subject Selection. Four families whose elders would otherwise have required nursing facility care participated in the study. These families consisted of all of the families within a six-month period who had contracted with the manufacturer to arrange installation of a Homecare Suite. The families were informed by the manufacturer about their opportunity to take part in a University research project. Names have been changed to protect the participants' identities.

Interviews. The Homecare Suite occupants and their family caregivers took part in at least two in-depth interviews consisting of a battery of rating scales, open-ended questions, and observations designed to learn about the older person's level of disability, social networks, affect, mental state, use of support services, housing satisfaction, living costs, family relationships and caregiver burden.

Homecare Suite Characteristics. The Homecare Suite consists of an accessible bedroom (standard unit, 12′ x 18′) and bathroom designed to meet the needs of frail occupants and their caregivers. The modular design allows the Suite to be custom-fit to nearly any size attached garage–including a single-car garage. Installation and removal of the Suite can usually be accomplished within 48 hours. The Suite attaches to the adjoining home's electrical system and contains a heat pump for heat and air conditioning, a water heater, and insulation. Plumbing and waste disposal systems are attached to the adjoining home's systems without major modifications. Figure 1 shows a typical floor plan.

The front facade (see Figure 2), which takes the place of the garage door, consists of siding customized to match the home, windows and

FIGURE 1

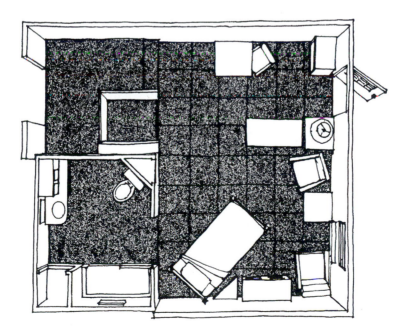

FIGURE 2

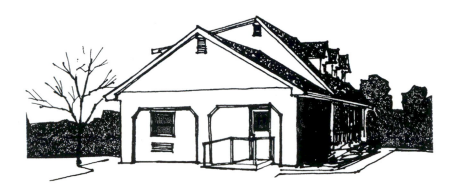

an outside door with a wheelchair ramp. A ramp or wheelchair elevator (depending on space and client wishes) leads to an interior door
into the adjoining home. A number of safety and accessibility features
are included, such as fire sprinklers, non-skid flooring, grab bars,
pull-out shelves, and a special slide-in bathtub to promote independent
bathing and eliminate caregiver lifting. An intercom allows communication from the Suite to the adjoining home.

While prices may vary by distributor, the purchase price in Kansas
of the Homecare Suite is $30,000. Alternatively, the units can be
rented on a month-to-month basis for $995 or leased for $499 (seven-
year lease) to $761 (one-year lease). Under a demonstration grant
funded by the Department of Housing and Urban Development, low-
income elders may rent the unit as a form of Section 8 housing.

To provide a basis for comparison, the average monthly Medicaid
rate for a nursing facility bed in Kansas is approximately $1,697, and
the average private pay rate is $1,815. Thus, the Homecare Suite rents
for around half the average cost of a nursing facility bed. The cost of
the Homecare Suite, however, does not include the cost of care, food,
or utilities.

CASE STUDIES

Table 1 provides a summary of demographic and background information for each of the participating families.

TABLE 1. Demographic Summary of Participating Families

	Family A	Family B	Family C	Family D
Age of User	87	83	79	79
Gender	Male	Female	Female	Female
Marital Status	Married	Widowed	Divorced	Widowed
User's Annual Income	$13,000 (includes wife)	$21,600	$15,000	$15,500
Health Status/ Disability	Bedfast; cognitive impairment	Had stroke; uses wheelchair	Mild dementia; uses wheel-chair	Moderate dementia; good mobility
Housing Prior to Suite Use	Hospital; skilled nursing facility	Hospital; nursing facility	Hospital; skilled nursing facility; daughter's dining room	Assisted living facility; daughter's living room
Primary Caregiver Demo-graphics	Daughter, 47, married, grown children	Daughter, 60, married, grown children	Daughter, 48, married, grown children	Daughter, 52 divorced, grown children
Caregiver's Annual Income	$30,000	$35,000	$60,000	$2,400
Home Occupants	Wife; Daughter and Son-in-law	Daughter and Son-in-law	Daughter and Son-in-law	Daughter; great-grand-daughter
Home Location	Small town	Large city	Mid-sized city	Mid-sized city
Home Accessibility	One level home but bathroom and doorways too small	One level home but bedrooms and bath inaccessible	Two level home; inaccessible bedrooms and bathrooms	One level home but bathroom diffi-cult to use
Where Would Person Have Lived Without Suite?	In nursing facility	In nursing facility	In nursing facility	In nursing facility

Family A: Mr. A, age 87, is a married, retired, white male who lives in a small midwestern town. Mr. A and his wife lived independently in their single-family home for forty years. In spring of 1993, Mr. A broke his hip and was in the hospital for 34 days. Because Mr. A's home was not accessible to someone with limited mobility, the family needed to find alternate housing for Mr. A. Alice, Mr. A's daughter, knew that if Mr. A were placed in a nursing facility, her parents would be terribly distressed by the separation, and her mother, who has a serious heart condition, would endanger her health by trying to visit Mr. A as often as possible. Alice wanted her parents to move in with her, but her house was too small and inaccessible to someone with a mobility impairment.

To solve the need for additional, accessible space, Alice decided to install a Homecare Suite in her single-car garage. Mr. A moved into the Homecare Suite, while Mrs. A moved into a bedroom in Alice's home. Mrs. A also used the Suite bathroom because it was easier and safer for her to do so. Mr. A received assistance during the day from a nurse's aide for 30 hours a week. Alice provided the rest of his care herself with some help from her mother and her two adult children. Alice reported that the hardest part about having her father at home was the loss of sleep and late nights. She estimated that she spent up to 70 hours per week involved in her father's care.

Alice was very pleased with the Homecare Suite and called it "year 2000 health care." She was satisfied with every aspect of the Suite, recommending it highly to others. The home-health aides were also very pleased with the Suite and the way it simplified caregiving. Alice estimated that her father's living costs, including rent, food, utilities, and health care, were about $1800 per month. This amount was about the same as what they would have paid for a room in a nursing facility, although Alice felt that the quality of care he was receiving in the Homecare Suite was much better.

A follow-up interview was conducted ten months after the Homecare Suite was installed. Alice's satisfaction remained high. She stressed that this option had allowed her to deal much more effectively with her father's health problems than otherwise would have been possible. For example, Alice reported that the special bathtub was extremely important in preventing pressure ulcers. Alice repeatedly said that keeping her parents at home extended both the length and quality of their lives. Alice also said that she gained peace of mind from knowing that her parents were receiving the best possible care in a home setting where they could be together. Alice reported having a lot less time to herself and a lot less privacy since she began using the Homecare Suite. She indicated, however, that she would have felt even more burdened if her father were in a nursing facility.

Family B: Mrs. B is an 83-year-old white female who lives in a large midwestern city. After her husband's death in 1989, she lived in a senior apartment complex for four years until she had a stroke. After a two-week hospital stay, she moved to a nursing facility where she lived for two months in a semiprivate room

Mrs. B's daughter, Barbara, is a 60-year-old college-educated homemaker who lives with her husband in a single-family home in the suburbs of the same city. Barbara served as her mother's primary caregiver since her father's death. Barbara was very dissatisfied with the care her mother was receiving at the nursing facility and was making three daily trips to supervise her mother's care. Barbara soon decided that she would prefer to care for her mother at her own home. Because Barbara's home was not wheelchair accessible, the Family decided to install a Homecare Suite in the home's double-car garage.

Once the Suite was installed, Barbara provided most of her mother's care. A private bath aide came two hours a day, five days a week, and Barbara received two hours of respite care each week through the Red Cross. Barbara estimated her mother's monthly living costs were about $1500, including the costs of rent, utilities, food, and the bath aide, compared to $2400 in the nursing facility.

Mrs. B responded that she was very satisfied with her living situation. The main reason she listed for wanting to use the Homecare Suite was so she could be close to her daughter. She said she couldn't think of any drawbacks, and she said she would recommend the Suite to others. Mrs. B rated her health as "very good" while she was in the nursing facility and "very good" while she was living in the Suite.

Barbara also said that she was very pleased with the Homecare Suite and reported that the Suite had been very helpful in meeting her mother's housing needs. Barbara said she would definitely recommend the Homecare Suite to others and that she would consider living in a Homecare Suite herself if she ever needed housing assistance.

Mrs. B and Barbara were interviewed again after they had been using the Homecare Suite for four months. Both reported that they continued to be very satisfied with the Suite and felt that it was meeting their needs very well. Barbara continued to spend about 70 hours per week in caregiving activities and reported that her role as primary caregiver was sometimes difficult. However, she stressed repeatedly that she much preferred to care for her mother at home where she could provide her with the best care possible.

Family C: Mrs. C, age 79, is a divorced, fully retired, white female who lived alone for forty years with only minimal contact with her family. In August of 1993, Mrs. C was hospitalized for malnutrition, dehydration and pancreatitis. After three weeks in the hospital she was moved to a skilled nursing facility for five weeks. Mrs. C suffered from depression, dementia, and a number of physical problems that her daughter, Cathy, believed would only improve if her mother were in a home-like setting under the careful supervision of relatives. Cathy's home, however, is not fully accessible to someone with limited mobility. The bedrooms are on the second level and there are other impediments such as small bathrooms and thick carpeting. While the family looked into housing options, Mrs. C lived in a temporary bedroom set up in the dining room on the first floor of Cathy's home. This arrangement was awkward and didn't provide either party with sufficient privacy. Delivering care was also difficult because the small bathroom on the first floor did not easily accommodate two people. In addition, Mrs. C had to be given bed-baths because the home's bathing facilities were not accessible to her. While living in the converted dining room, Mrs. C tripped on the carpeting and had to be hospitalized for eleven days for a broken hip and dislocated shoulder.

The Homecare Suite was installed during Mrs. C's hospitalization. Upon return home, her care was provided by a combination of visiting nurses and private personal-care aides for forty hours per week. A private aide also came once every other week for four hours in the evening. Cathy and her husband provided care in the evening and on weekends.

Mrs. C reported that she was quite pleased with living in a Homecare Suite and would recommend it to others. Mrs. C weighed 65 lbs. when she arrived from the nursing facility. After living in the Homecare Suite for one month, her weight increased to 77 lbs. Cathy rated her mother's health as "fair" before moving into the Suite, and "good" after the move.

Cathy was quite pleased with having added a Homecare Suite to her home and said that the Suite had been very helpful in meeting her mother's housing needs. Cathy listed the ability to provide high quality care and the ease of delivering personal care as being the two main reasons that she wanted to continue using the Homecare Suite. The Visiting Nurses were also very supportive of the Homecare Suite because it made caregiving easier. Cathy estimated that her mother's living costs (including Suite rental food, utilities, and health care) totaled $1500 per month, while the alternatives they had considered ranged from $2000 to $3000.

Cathy noted that caring for her mother had been stressful. She estimated that she spent at least 52 hours per week involved in her mother's care. She rated this level of involvement as "too much" but felt it was necessary to maintain her mother's health and well-being. However, Cathy said that she would recommend the Homecare Suite to others and that she would consider living in a Homecare Suite herself if she ever needed housing assistance.

Cathy and Mrs. C participated in a follow-up interview four months after installing the Homecare Suite. Both reported that the Suite continued to be very helpful in meeting their housing needs. Mrs. C's physical health continued to improve, as shown by her weight gain to 85 lbs. at the time of the third interview. This change was reflected in Mrs. C's own assessment of her health, which went from "good" at the second interview to "very good" at the third.

Family D: Mrs. D is a 79-year-old retired, white female who had lived independently in a small midwestern town since her husband's death in 1952. In 1993 she started to show some signs of dementia. Mrs. D moved to a retirement complex with independent apartments but was asked to leave within two weeks because she required too much care. Mrs. D then moved into a semi-private room in an assisted living facility. Alter one month, she was asked to leave because of her nocturnal wandering.

Mrs. D's daughter, Dana, had made multiple daily trips to the assisted living facility. She decided it would be easier and less expensive to care for her mother at home. Dana, age 54, is divorced and lives in a small (875 square feet) two-bedroom modular home with her granddaughter, age 10. Because she didn't have an extra bedroom for her mother, Dana turned her living room into a temporary bedroom. The small bathroom, with its traditional bathtub and shower, was difficult for Mrs. D to use. Alter five weeks, the family decided to install a Homecare Suite in the home's single-car garage.

Dana provided all of her mother's care except for 5 hours of daily help from a private aide. Because of Mrs. D wandering, they installed a security system with buzzers on the doors. The door from the Suite into the main home was cut in half so that the bottom part of the door could be secured to prevent wandering but the top could be opened to allow supervision.

Mrs. D said she was very pleased with living in a Homecare Suite and she noted that one of the main benefits of the Suite was the independence it gave her, allowing her to "be my own boss." Dana was also very satisfied with her mother's living situation and felt that the Homecare Suite was very helpful in meeting her mother's housing needs. She noted that the move was not at all stressful for her mother and only slightly stressful for her. The main reason Dana wanted to continue using the Suite was to be able to provide Mrs. D with the best care possible. Dana said that she would recommend the Suite to others and would consider living in a Homecare Suite if she ever needed housing assistance. Dana estimated that her mother's monthly living costs totaled $1925, while the assisted living facility was $2550 per month.

Dana noted that Mrs. D was much calmer and more alert since moving into the Homecare Suite, to the point that her dementia medication had been discontinued. While Mrs. D previously wandered several times per night, her nocturnal wandering became rare after moving into the Homecare Suite. Dana rated her mother's health as "very good" before moving into the Suite, and "excellent" after the move.

DISCUSSION

The results of this preliminary evaluation offer substantial grounds for optimism. The Homecare Suite received endorsement from all users and their caregivers. All the families reported that the cost of the Suite was reasonable. Families and users reported that they had more privacy than would otherwise have been possible in a home-sharing situation. At the same time, families found that the proximity of the Suite, along with the special accessibility features, made it easier to provide care. Similarly, Homecare Suites were viewed by service providers as facilitating the provision of care. Indeed, satisfaction by all of the participants was uniformly high.

One concern raised by this study and by a market study of the Homecare Suite (see Mathews, Altus & Kosloski, 1994) was the large amount of time spent by family members in caregiving tasks. Families interested in using the Homecare Suite should be assisted by a social worker to obtain outside caregiver assistance and respite care to meet their needs.

For families who want to care for their elders but whose homes are too small or inaccessible, the Homecare Suite offers an option previously unavailable. The population for whom this option is suited may be small, but the potential savings to families and the state, in both human and monetary costs, may be substantial. This study suggests that the Homecare Suite is deserving of further study on a larger scale.

REFERENCES

AARP. (1988). ECHO: A housing option waiting to happen. *AARP Housing Report*, August/September, 1-6.

Lazarowich, N. M. (1991). *Granny Flats as Housing for the Elderly: International Perspectives.* New York: The Haworth Press, Inc.

Mathews, R M., Altus, D. E., & Kosloski, K D. (1994). *Market analysis of an accessible housing option for disabled elders.* Paper presented at the annual conference of the Gerontological Society of America, Atlanta, GA.

Index

FORTHCOMING and NEW BOOKS FROM HAWORTH AGING, GERONTOLOGY & LONG-TERM CARE

MAKING AGING IN PLACE WORK
NEW!

Edited by Leon A. Pastalan, PhD
Helps social workers and family members of elderly individuals improve the quality of life for loved ones by enabling the aging to stay in their current living arrangement for as long as possible.
(A monograph published simultaneously as the Journal of Housing for the Elderly, Vol. 16, No. 4.)
$39.95 hard. ISBN: 0-7890-0753-3.
Text price (5+ copies): $24.95.
Available Summer 1999. Approx. 145 pp. with Index.

FUNDAMENTALS OF FEMINIST GERONTOLOGY
NEW!

Edited by J. Dianne Garner, DSW
This book strives to increase women's self-esteem and their overall quality of life by encouraging education and putting a stop to age, sex, and race discrimination.
(A monograph published simultaneously as the Journal of Women & Aging, Vol. 11, No. 2/3.)
$39.95 hard. ISBN: 0-7890-0761-4.
$24.95 soft. ISBN: 0-7890-0762-2.
Available Summer 1999. Approx. 200 pp. with Index.

ELDER ABUSE AND NEGLECT IN RESIDENTIAL SETTINGS
NEW!

Different National Backgrounds and Similar Responses
Edited by Frank Glendenning, PhD, and Paul Kingston, PhD
Gain insights from countries where elder abuse and neglect have been recognized as an issue requiring social policy attention.
(A monograph published simultaneously as Journal of Elder Abuse & Neglect, Vol. 10, No. 1/2.)
$39.95 hard. ISBN: 0-7890-0751-7.
Text price (5+ copies): $24.95.
Available Spring 1999. Approx. 204 pp. with Index.

DIABETES MELLITUS IN THE ELDERLY

Edited by James W. Cooper, PharmPhD
NEW!
Keeps you up-to-date with the latest information concerning the treatment and understanding of conditions that lead to diabetes mellitus.
(A monograph published simultaneously as the Journal of Geriatric Drug Therapy, Vol. 12, No. 2.)
$39.95 hard. ISBN: 0-7890-0682-0.
Text price (5+ copies): $24.95.
1999. Available now. 121 pp. with Index.

Textbooks are available for classroom adoption consideration on a 60-day examination basis. You will receive an invoice payable within 60 days along with the book. **If you decide to adopt the book, your invoice will be cancelled.** Please write to us on your institutional letterhead, indicating the textbook you would like to examine as well as the following information: course title, current text, enrollment, and decision date.

LATINO ELDERS AND THE TWENTY-FIRST CENTURY
NEW!

Issues and Challenges for Culturally Competent Research and Practice
Edited by Melvin Delgado, PhD
This book will help you develop and create culturally competent intervention methods that take the culture, beliefs, and situations of Latino elders into consideration.
(A monograph published simultaneously as the Journal of Gerontological Social Work, Vol. 30, Nos. 1/2.)
$49.95 hard. ISBN: 0-7890-0657-X.
Text price (5+ copies): $29.95.
1999. Available now. 207 pp. with Index.

GRIEF EDUCATION FOR CAREGIVERS OF THE ELDERLY
NEW!

Junietta Baker McCall, DMin
It is filled with stories from elderly persons and from those who care for them. You'll find numerous suggestions for improving your efforts to help aging and dying elderly persons.
$49.95 hard. ISBN: 0-7890-0498-4.
Text price (5+ copies): $29.95.
1999. Available now. 190 pp. with Index.
Features case studies, workshop creation handouts and examples, figures, and a bibliography.

FULL CIRCLE
NEW!

Spiritual Therapy for the Elderly
Kevin Kirkland and Howard McIlveen, MDiv
Over 200 Pages!
Discover a brand new therapeutic approach—spiritual therapy—to treating elderly patients with cognitive disorders. This handy guide will guide you in starting your own renowned spiritually therapeutic program for dementia patients.
$29.95 hard. ISBN: 0-7890-0606-5.
Text price (5+ copies): $14.95.
1999. Available now. 235 pp. with 2 Indexes.
Features lists of hymns, prayers, songs, and poetry.

PREPARING PARTICIPANTS FOR INTERGENERATIONAL INTERACTION
NEW!

Training for Success
Edited by Melissa O. Hawkins, MS, Kenneth F. Backman, PhD, and Francis A. McGuire, PhD
Contains exercises that will help you train colleagues and volunteers for these specific programs and includes criteria for activity evaluations.
(A monograph published simultaneously as Activities, Adaptation & Aging, Vol. 23, Nos. 1/2/3.)
$39.95 hard. ISBN: 0-7890-0367-8.
Text price (5+ copies): $24.95
1999. Available now. 196 pp. with Index.

The Haworth Press, Inc.
10 Alice Street, Binghamton New York 13904-1580 USA

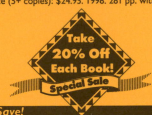

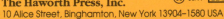